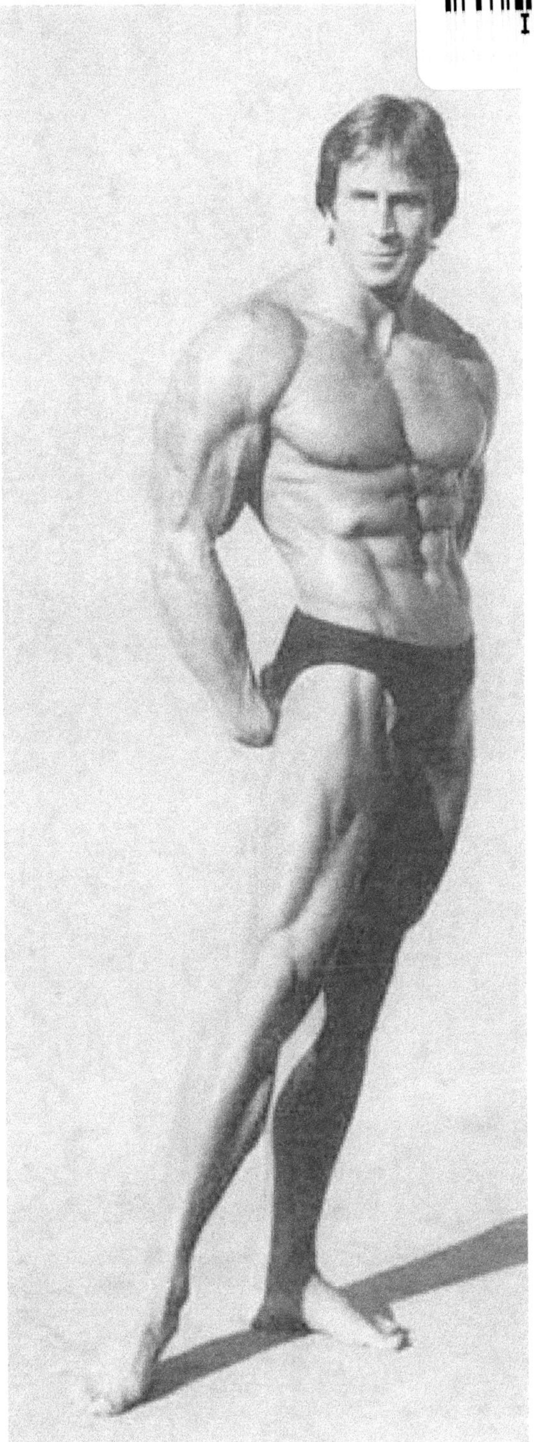

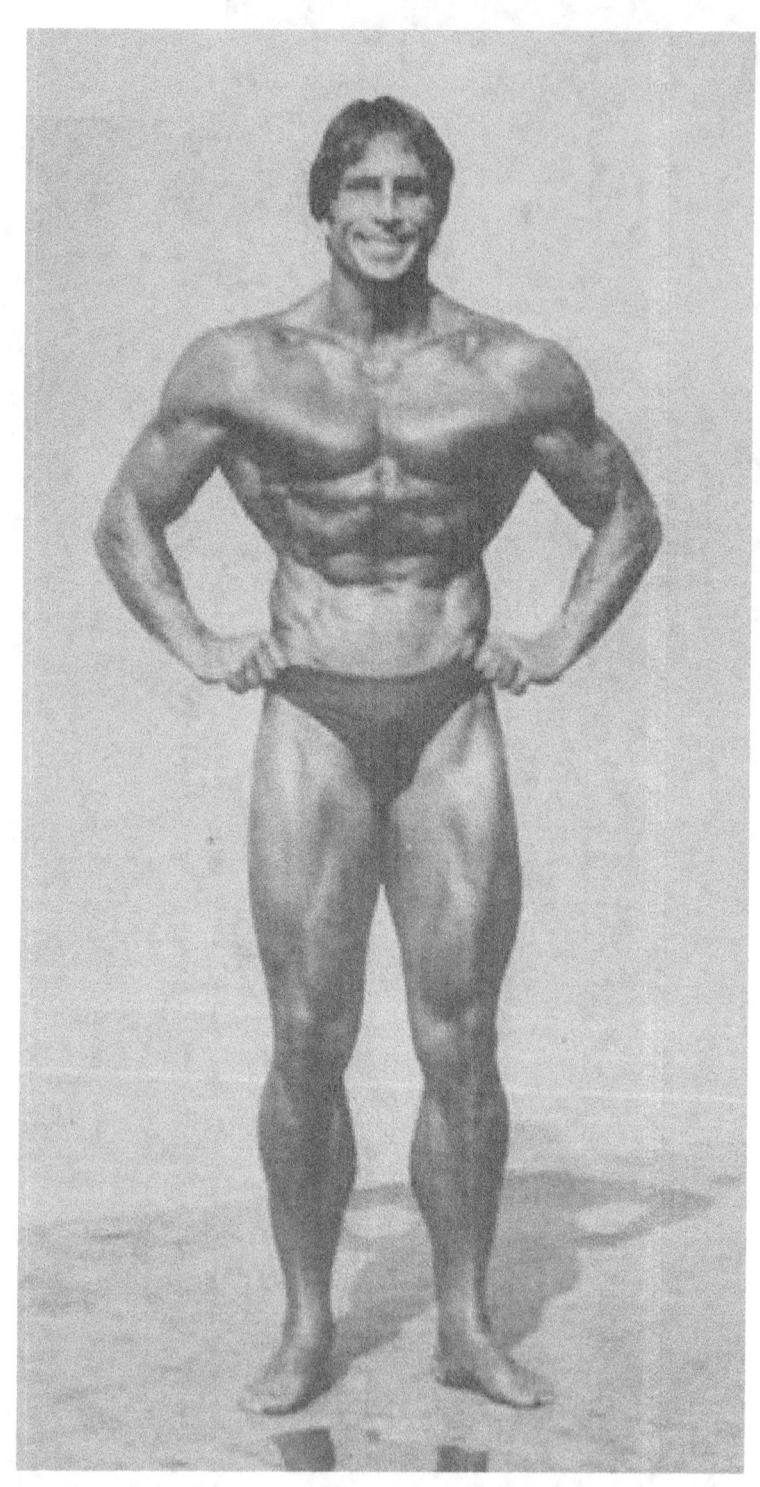

the magic of SYMMETRY

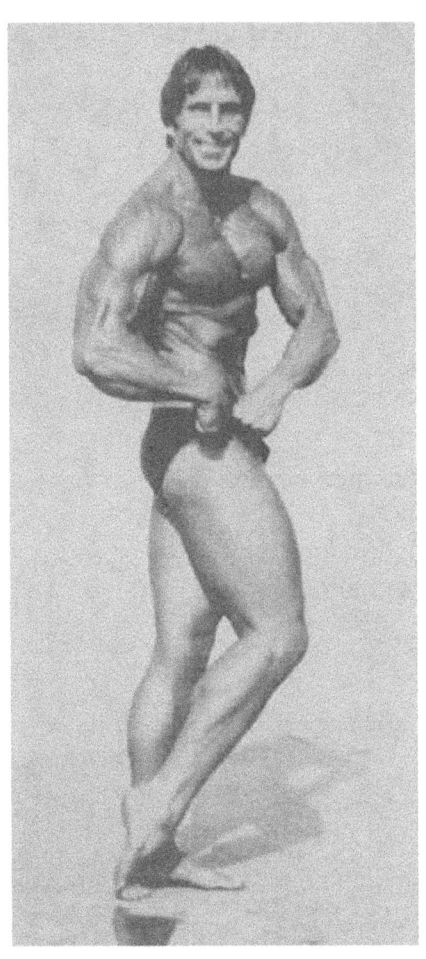

by Steve Davis

The Magic of Symmetry
By Steve Davis

First Edition 1976
Second Edition 2014

ISBN-13: 978-1502797735
ISBN-10: 1502797739

Published by:
Steve Davis 2355 Westwood Blvd. #570
Los Angeles, CA. 90064-2109
www.SteveDavisBodybuilder.com
Email: SteveDavisBodybuilder@yahoo.com

Also by Steve Davis, <u>Achieving Total Muscularity</u>

This book is dedicated to Pamela, my source of inspiration.

Table of Contents

Foreword

by Harvey Keith

We have called this particular thesis The Magic of Symmetry for a very specific reason. Aesthetically, the symmetrical physique is incomparable. When one of the few bodybuilders of our era who possess this elusive quality, steps on the stage, the audience seems to be held spellbound! It has an almost magical or hypnotic effect on even the untrained eye of a non-bodybuilder or female fan. It is this charisma that can allow a smaller yet more symmetrical physique competitor to beat men far heavier or larger than himself. Steve Davis has proven this time and again in competition.

We believe that it is the various specific qualities that, in total, we have come to call symmetry that will determine the "New Breed" of physique champion. He will be a man unconcerned with freaky body parts or size for the sake of mere size. His will be the thickly muscled yet pleasing body of the 21st Century. At one time, the word symmetry meant an evenly developed physique all around. This concept gained popularity at the turn of the century with the immense fame of "the father of modern bodybuilding," Eugen Sandow. For decades, the "authorities" in our sport believed a symmetrical physique had to have neck, calf and arm measurements that were exactly equal. Certainly by today's bodybuilding criteria this would be impossible. Then, one must ask himself what are the magical qualities that comprise the physique of the New Breed of champion?

Symmetry has come to mean something quite different than in Sandow's day. First, the taper or differential between the shoulder width and hip-waist area is of paramount importance. The degree of muscularity and definition has also become a part of the quality we now call symmetry. The shape of each of the various muscle groups and their proportion to each other has become relevant. Vascularity has become an intrinsic factor in the new concept of symmetry. Even skin tone is important. The total sum of all these aforementioned, difficult to attain, attributes is what comprises the magic of symmetry. If a bodybuilder has truly

1

captured these elusive qualities he will generate an amazing amount of charisma whether he steps upon the posing dais or on to the beach.

About the Author

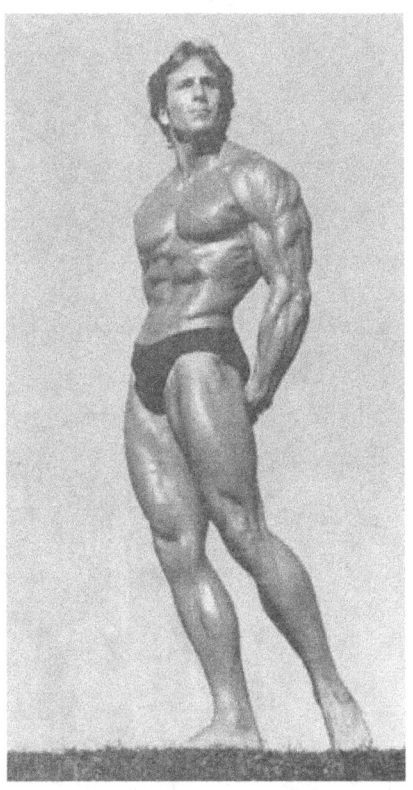

Steve Davis-Once weighed over 285 pounds! Through an original and innovative program of progressive resistance exercise and scientific nutrition, Steve was able to lose over 100 pounds to win the Mr. California title. His miraculous transformation has rendered him one of the most sought after physical culture and nutritional science authorities in the country.

The Symmetrical Ideal

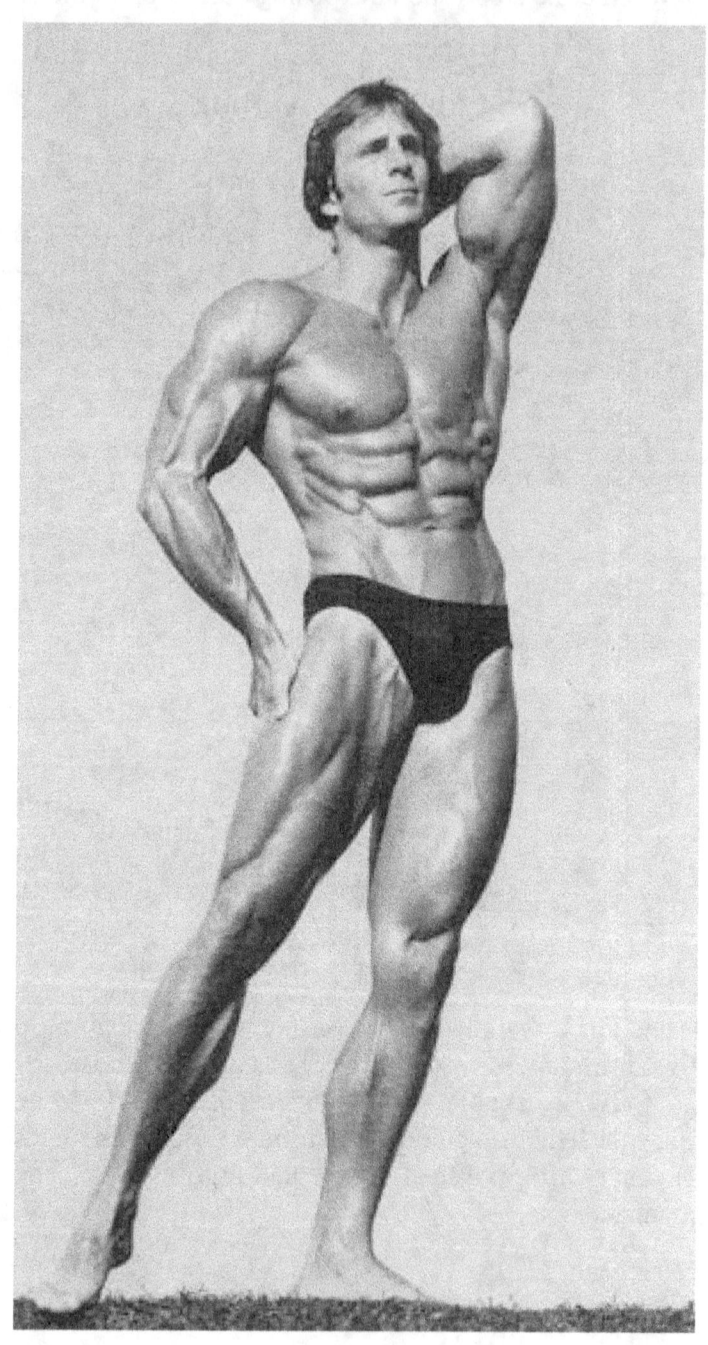

The Symmetrical Ideal

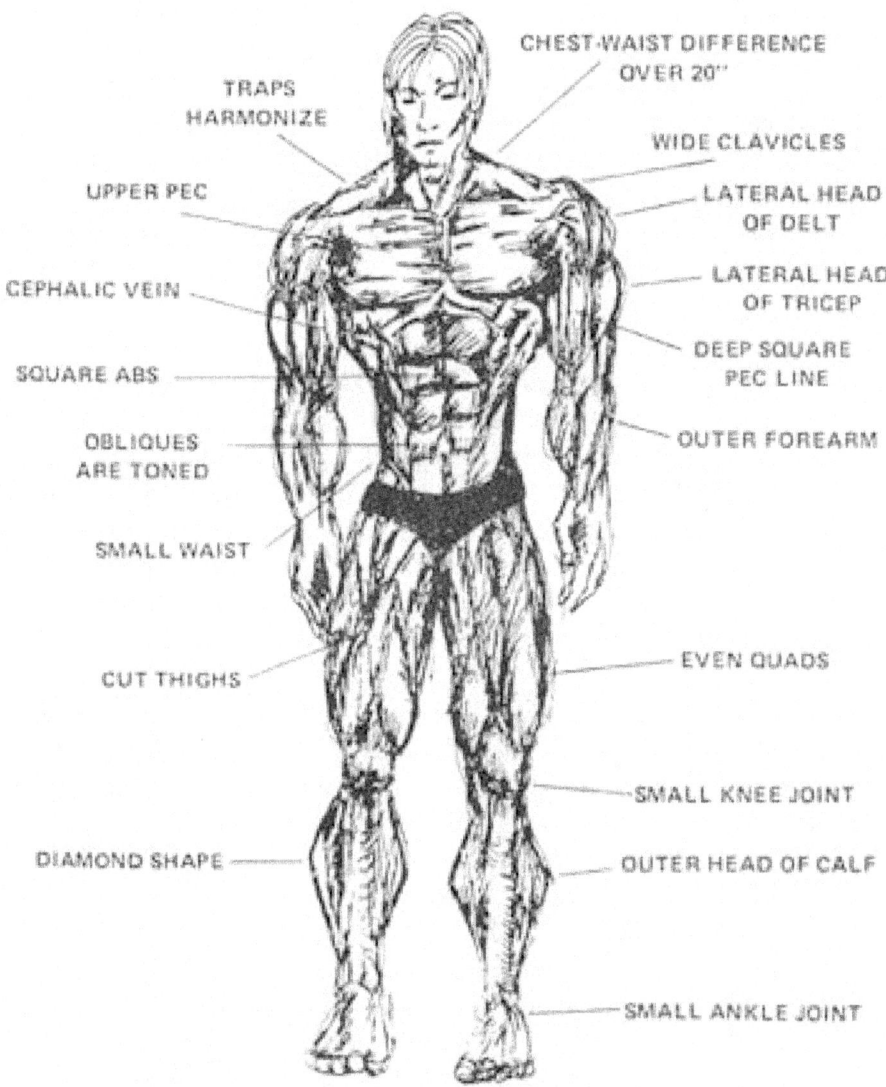

TRAPS HARMONIZE

UPPER PEC

CEPHALIC VEIN

SQUARE ABS

OBLIQUES ARE TONED

SMALL WAIST

CUT THIGHS

DIAMOND SHAPE

CHEST-WAIST DIFFERENCE OVER 20"

WIDE CLAVICLES

LATERAL HEAD OF DELT

LATERAL HEAD OF TRICEP

DEEP SQUARE PEC LINE

OUTER FOREARM

EVEN QUADS

SMALL KNEE JOINT

OUTER HEAD OF CALF

SMALL ANKLE JOINT

LOWER BODY AS DEVELOPED AS UPPER

4

The Symmetrical Ideal

Before seeking to attain a symmetrical physique the trainee must know exactly what he is striving for. The optimum symmetrical physique is one of varied qualities. As mentioned in the foreword the first outstanding quality to be considered is maximum shoulder and waist differential. The deltoids should be developed to the fullest with a squareness achieved by special emphasis on development of the lateral head (side delt). The trapezius should not be overly full. The pectorals should be as square as possible (this is determined by heredity). The delineation of these large chest muscles should be deeply etched. The pectoralis minor (upper pec) should be developed to its limit. The major or lower pec should not be overdone. The line between the two pectorals should be striated and defined.

The arms should be slightly out of proportion to the rest of the physique. Just a bit too big for everything else. All three heads of the triceps should be developed with cross striations throughout the muscle. Special attention should be placed on the lateral (outer) head and the low tricep (length of tricep is also a function of heredity). The biceps should have both heads developed equally with plenty of low bicep and peak. Maximum development of the cephalic vein that runs down the biceps is also to be considered. The forearms should be full and very vascular with equal development of inner and outer musculature.

The thighs should be evenly developed with both quadriceps muscles over the knee as square and evenly matched as possible. Deep cuts in the thigh are a must. The side of the thigh must have as deep a cut as possible between the front thigh muscles and the leg biceps. There should be a good degree of sweep on the side of thigh tapering down to a small knee.

The calf should be diamond shaped and low. This diamond should taper down from a small knee joint to a proportionately small ankle. From the rear, the calf should be split and evenly developed from both sides. Deep cuts should accent the outer heads of the gastrocnemius and soleus. The leg biceps should be as muscular as possible. This long muscle should be tapered and sweep from the base of a small, but muscular gluteus maximus (buttocks) to the back of the knee. The gluteus should tie in nicely with thickly developed and cross striated erectors. The obliques should be muscular but seem underdeveloped comparatively. The latissimus should be built to their fullest. The rear trapezius should be thick and will defined. Deltoids should tie in with proportionately less developed upper traps. The biceps should show good peak from the rear.

Remember, you can never have shoulders that are too wide. Your arms cannot be overdone if proper balance between biceps and triceps is maintained. The erectors cannot be too thick. The upper pec cannot be overdeveloped. No one ever exhibited too big a calf. The thigh can never be too cut up. Maintain as dazzling a taper as possible. The other muscle groups can be overdone. Keep this in mind and picture the symmetrical ideal as you train.

Achieving the Symmetrical Ideal

There is a master template for your physique. Each major body part has an optimum shape, that when combined, creates an illusion that the entire physique is much greater than the sum of its composite parts.
Beginning with the calves, both the gastrocnemius (upper calf) and the soleus (lower calf) should harmonize. Many trainees neglect the soleus and end up with what is commonly referred to as a high calf. Development of the soleus also produces the much desired diamond-shape.

The muscle complex of the frontal thigh must be balanced with an equal amount of leg bicep. Most physique competitors can hide faulty leg biceps in their front poses, but when viewed from the side or rear, weak femoral biceps can be a devastating blow to any upper body. Besides a balanced front and rear thigh, the upper and lower width differential of the thigh should be as small as possible. Don't mistake small knees and small lower thighs as equally desirable.

Over development of the abdominals can ruin your body. True as this statement is, I still see some aspiring trainees doing weighted sidebends. Forget your obliques! Never train them. Instead, concentrate on equal work for the upper and lower abdominals. Most ab exercises work the upper two-thirds of the abdominal cavity, leaving the lower region smooth and fatty. Unfortunately, many so-called lower ab movements hit only the upper two rows.

The rib cage can only be developed if you are wide enough at the shoulders to handle it. The day of the barrel chest is gone forever. The chest-heavy syndrome goes as follows: heavy squats and pullovers are done to gain weight by the young enthusiast. Then, since nothing looks worse than a big rib cage and small pecs, the trainee does countless sets of bench presses. Finally, the pecs do catch up with the rib cage, but by then, the chances of having WIDE shoulders is all but hereditarily impossible.

The pectorals are basically dual-muscle structures. The pectoral major (lower pec) comprises 75% and is many times easier to develop than the pectoral minor (upper pec) which is only 25% of the total area. The problem is obvious. The lower pecs must be contained as you perform twice as much work for the upper pecs. Face it, gravity is against you. Concentrate on upper pec work.

The shoulders must never be confused with the trapezius muscles. Deltoids are usually weak in the lateral (side) and posterior (rear) regions. Pressing movements contribute almost entirely to the anterior (frontal) deltoid so that the chances of underdeveloped anterior deltoids is almost impossible. For shoulder width, train the lateral head of the deltoid mercilessly. To ensure that your upper back is explosive, blast the posterior heads. Remember, the lateral and posterior heads of the deltoid can never be overdeveloped! The trapezius muscles should be trained a total of 10% of your deltoid work. Don't ruin your natural width by developing a sloping-trap-heavy-shoulder complex. I train my traps about 30 days a year. Sometimes.

Symmetrical biceps consist of achieving low bicep attachment and a peaking outer head simultaneously. Most bodybuilders I instruct have one of the above ingredients and are usually in the process of obtaining the other. Naturally, the realization that there are two major areas of emphasis when considering this area simplifies your training procedure immensely. I only wish someone would have suggested this to me years ago. Anyway, I'm glad that those of you who are willing can benefit from my experience.

I personally think very few men possess proportionate triceps. You must strive to produce a tricep that begins as close as anatomically feasible to the elbow joint. Also, of the three heads, more emphasis should be placed on creating a very muscular outside head. Remember, both the biceps and triceps can never be overdeveloped. (Can you imagine any of us being so lucky?)

The forearms must harmonize with the size of your arms--specifically the lower biceps. My forearms are large enough and respond fast from any movement that requires a grip, so I don't need to train them directly. To create harmony from the deltoid to the hands, the forearms must complement the arms, not compete with them for size impressiveness.

Even though many trainees consider their lats to be well developed, only a few men meet the requirements of a truly symmetrical back. Equal emphasis must be placed on all three sections of the back. Besides the upper back, or lats, there is a middle and lower portion, all demanding balance of development.

I call the erector muscles the missing link between the upper and lower body. I can remember only a few trainees doing any kind of direct erector exercise. And yet, moderate development of this muscle group will make the lower two-thirds of the back look finished, rather than like the just-out-of-a-cast appearance.

Anatomical Self Analysis

Stand in front of a full length mirror in your posing trunks or bathing suit. Try to find a mirror with an overhead light. Position yourself so the shadow projected down from your nose hits the middle and lower pec lines. Stand completely relaxed. Be objective. How do you stack up to the symmetrical ideal discussed previously? Do you have mature, quality muscle? Make a mental note of your weak points. These are your targets for the next full year. Bringing them up to par is the only way to achieve the symmetry you desire. Check your physique for pockets of fat. For instance many trainees store fat in the pectorals or obliques. Just realistically follow the seven master steps to a symmetrical physique listed below and watch your physique begin to transform.

Step I   Stand in front of a mirror.

Step II   Be as objective as possible.

Step III Examine each of the ten body parts and calculate sectional (see Symmetrical Ideal) differences and record all areas that need improvement.

Step IV   Once you have the data on exactly what specific areas you need to emphasize, select the corresponding exercises in 'Correction of Weak Body Parts' and place them in one of the routine formations listed in the section 'Restructured Training.'

Step V   Stay on each program you create for 6 weeks - 12 weeks. Try a different combination of exercises within a given routine after reviewing steps I - IV.

Step VI   Have someone take black and white photos of you at the beginning and end of each program. Keep accurate pictorial records of your improvement.

Step VII Always seek to find what works for you and disregard what others are doing. No two men have the same bodies, therefore no two men respond the same.

Summary Chart Anatomical Self Analysis

Body Part	Anatomical Self Analysis (% Point of Emphasis)	Danger Area
1. Calf	50/50 balance between soleus and gastrocnemius	underdeveloped soleus
2. Thigh	60/40 balance between quadraceps and leg biceps	underdeveloped leg bicep
3. Abdominals	50/50 balance between upper and lower Ab's	never train obliques
4. Rib Cage	Developed only as shoulder width permits	"chest-heavy syndrome"
5. Pectorals	Seek to have more upper than lower pectoral	sagging lower pecs
6. Shoulders	Of total deltoid training time: 20% Anterior, 40% lateral, 40% posterior. (Note: only 10% of delt work should go towards the traps. (Example: If you do 20 sets for delts then 2 sets for traps!)	too much frontal delt and/or trapezius
7. Biceps	50/50 balance between low bicep and outer bicep peak	high bicep, or flat bicep
8. Triceps	50/50 balance between upper and lower tricep, then 30% more outside tricep work	high tricep, no outside tricep muscularity
9. Forearms	The width of the upper forearm should be 40% and the width of the lower bicep should be 60	over or underdeveloped forearms in comparison to upper arms
10a. Back	33 ⅓% balance between the three sections of the back: upper, mid and lower	usually, underdeveloped mid and lower back
10b. Erectors	Sufficient development to create a look of depth throughout the lower ⅔' s of the back	Minimal thickness

Restructured Training

By now you have recognized the deficient areas of your physique, and you want to begin correcting them. The concept of restructured training is a plan to place greater training emphasis on your weak body parts. I will list three different programs designed for this concentration.

Program I

This schedule is designed to bring as many as four deficient body parts up to par with the remainder of the physique, while still training the advanced muscle sections twice weekly. Using the suggested list of 10 possible body parts, here would be a typical example of a seven day a week routine for shoulder and arm specialization.

Monday-Friday
1. Chest
2. Back

Wednesday-Sunday
1. Thighs
2. Erectors
3. Abs
4. Calves

Tuesday- Thursday-Saturday *
1. Shoulders
2. Biceps
3. Triceps
4. Forearms

*(Note: This is only an example, you may substitute any weak body parts on these three days, but do not train any more than 4 body parts.

Program II

This schedule is for the trainee who can only train six days per week. Again, as in Program I up to 4 body parts maybe specialized on. Here is a sample routine for someone who wants to specialize on shoulders, back, biceps and calves.

Monday-Wednesday-Friday
1. Shoulders
2. Back
3. Biceps
4. Calves

Tuesday-Thursday-Saturday
1. Chest
2. Triceps
3. Forearms
4. Thighs
5. Erectors
6. Calves

For those trainees whose lower bodies are behind their upper bodies here is a 5 day a week routine that is most effective. This program can also be used by someone who wants to specialize but who can only train 5 days per week. (Note: This routine may be reversed to emphasize upper body development.)

Monday-Wednesday- Friday – Lower Body
1. Thighs
2. Calves
3. Erectors
4. Abs

Tuesday-Thursday – Upper Body
1. Chest
2. Back
3. Shoulders
4. Biceps
5. Triceps
6. Forearms

Correction of Weak Body Parts

To simplify your attempts at achieving a more symmetrical physique you should use this guide to zero-in on that section of your particular body part. Regarding sets and reps, I would say generally, 10-15 sets per body part, 5 sets per exercise, therefore, 2 - 3 exercises per body part, whether you are specializing on that area or not. The routines are designed to emphasize weak points, not by doing more sets and reps on a given day, but by increasing the days per week the area is worked. In this manner you will not over train the areas to be specialized on and at the same time not under train the contrasting body parts. Here is a rule of thumb for repetitions:

For calves, thighs, forearms and abdominals do 15 - 30.
For deltoids, biceps, triceps, pecs and the back complex do 8 - 12.

Body Parts and Corrective Exercises

1. CALVES
    a. Soleus
        1. Seated Calf Raise
        2. Leg Press Calf Raise
    b. Gastrocnemius
        1. Donkey Calf Raise
        2. Wall Calf Machine
        3. Press Machine Raise

2. THIGHS
    a. Rectus Femoris (lower front thigh above knee)
        1. Hack Squats
        2. Angle Squats
        3. Plié Squat
    b. Femoral Bicep (leg bicep)
        1. Leg Curl
        2. Upper extension
        3. Stiff legged dead lift

3. ABDOMINAL
    a. Upper Rectus Abdominis
        1. Crunch
        2. ¼ Sit Up
    b. Lower Rectus Abdominis
        1. Hanging Knee Up
        2. Lying Leg Raise

4. RIB CAGE
        1. One Dumbbell Pullover
        2. Barbell Pullover

5. PECTORALS
    a. Pectoral Minor (upper pec)
        1. Barbell Incline Press
        2. Dumbbell Incline Press
        3. Neck Press
    b. Pectoral Major (lower pec)
        1. Flat Bench Laterals
    c. Lower Pec Outline
        1. V-Bar Wide Dips
        2. Cable Crushes

6. DELTOIDS
    a. Anterior Head (decline front)
        1. Front Cable Raise
        2. Criss-Cross Barbell Raise
        3. Alternate Dumbbell Raise
    b. Lateral Head (side)
        1. Standing Dumbbell Raise
        2. Side Cable Raise
        3. Wide Upright Rows
        4. One Dumbbell Incline Raise
    c. Posterior Head (rear)
        1. Bent Over Laterals
        2. Bent Cable Cross-overs
        3. Face Down Lateral Raise

7. BICEPS
    a. Lower Bicep
        1. Preacher Curl
        2. Strict Barbell Curl
        3. Low Incline Dumbbell Curl
    b. Outer Peak
        1. Spider Curl
        2. Cable Curls
        3. Concentration Curl

8. TRICEPS

   a. Low Tricep
      1. Close Grip Bench Press
      2. Lying French Press
      3. Standing Cable Extension
      4. Standing French Press
      5. Dumbbell Decline French Press
   b. Outer Tricep Head (lateral head)
      1. Tricep Pull
      2. Pushdown
      3. Standing Cable Extension

9. FOREARMS

      1. Dead Stop Wrist Curl
      2. Reverse Wrist Curl
      3. High Rep Reverse Curls
      4. Reverse Preacher Curl

10. BACK

   a. Upper Back (Rhomboideus Major-Minor, Infra Spinatus, Terres Major-Minor)
      1. Wide Chins
      2. Wide Pulldowns
      3. Bent Over Laterals
   b. Middle Back (Latissimus Dorsi)
      1. Bent Over Rowing
      2. Leverage Rowing
      3. Long Pull
      4. Short Pull
   c. Lower Back (Erector)
      1. Hyperextensions
      2. Deadlift
      3. Good Mornings

The Optimum Torso

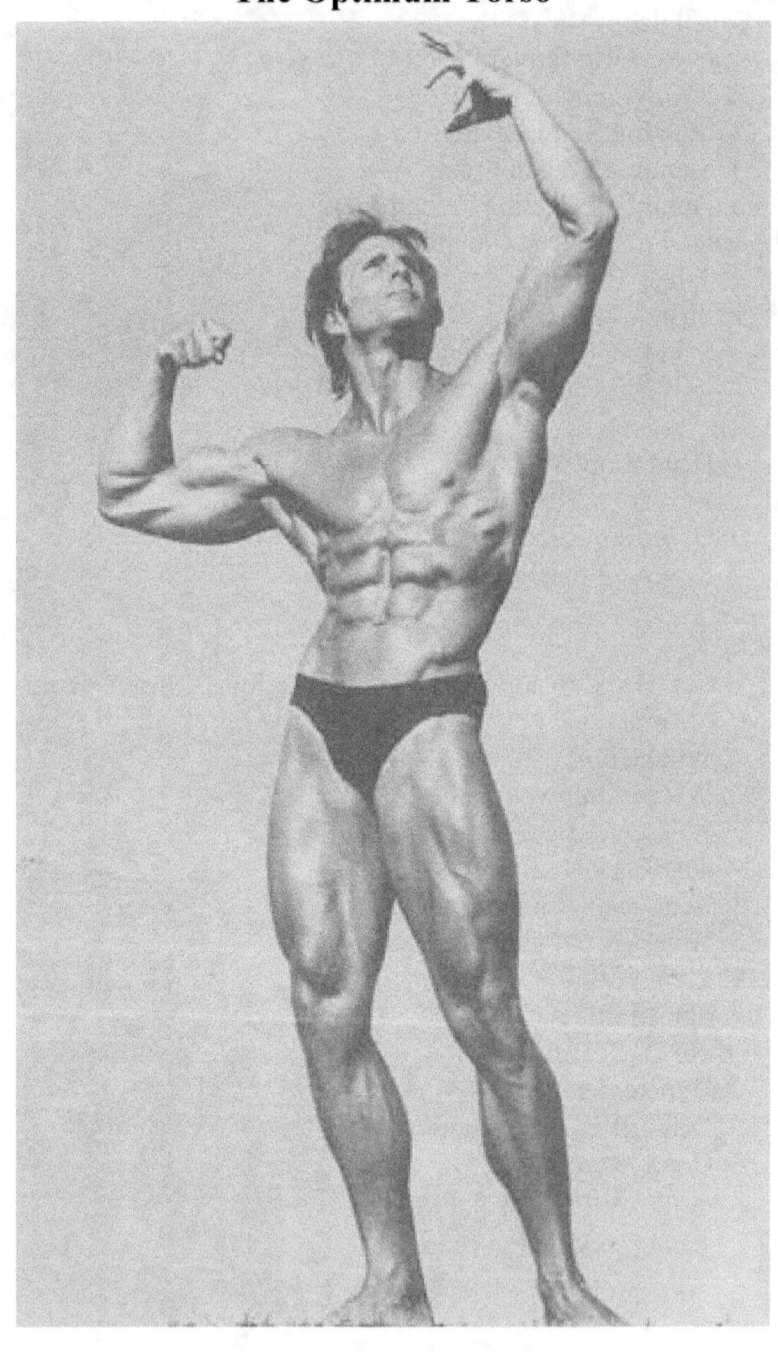

The Optimum Torso

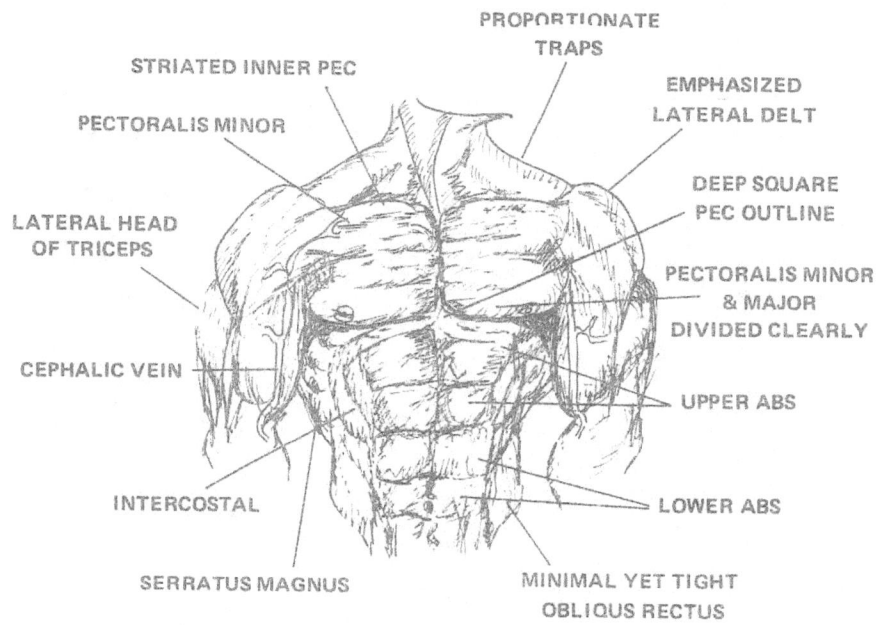

STRIATED INNER PEC- Close Grip Bench Press, Crushing Movements with cables, using a chest crusher, D.B. Incline Press.
PECTORALIS MINOR-Incline Press, Bench Press to neck.
PECTORAL Outline- V-Bar Dips, Dumbbell Flyes, D.B. Pullovers.
SERRATUS MAGNUS- D.B. Pullovers, Wide Chins, Lat Pulldowns.
DELINIATION BETWEEN PECTORALIS MAJOR & MINOR- V-Bar dips, Incline D.B. Flyes.
UPPER ABDOMINALS- Crunches, ¼ Sit Up.
LOWER ABDOMINALS- Hanging Knee Up. INTERCOSTALS- Pullover movements, Hanging Knee Up.
PECTORAL DELTOID TIE-IN- All flying movements, Dips, Pullovers, ⅔ Bench Press high on chest or neck, Incline Press.

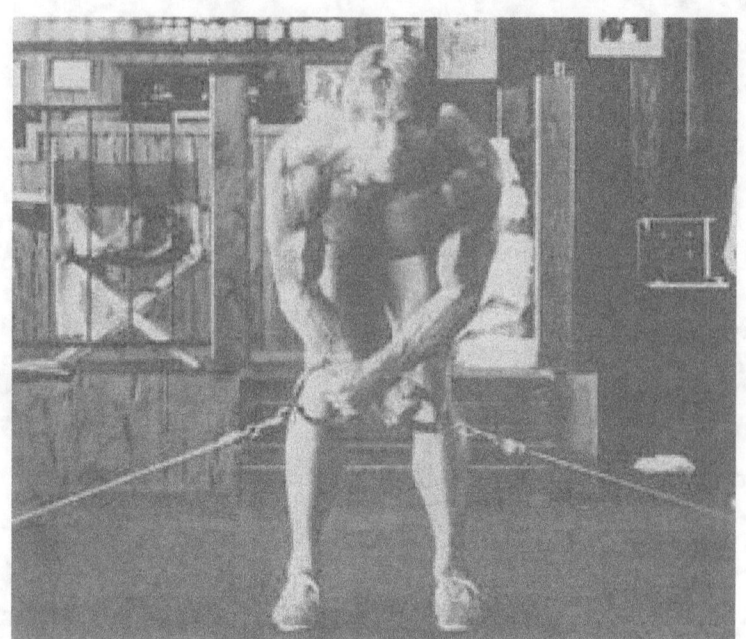

Pecs – Pulley Crushes (start)

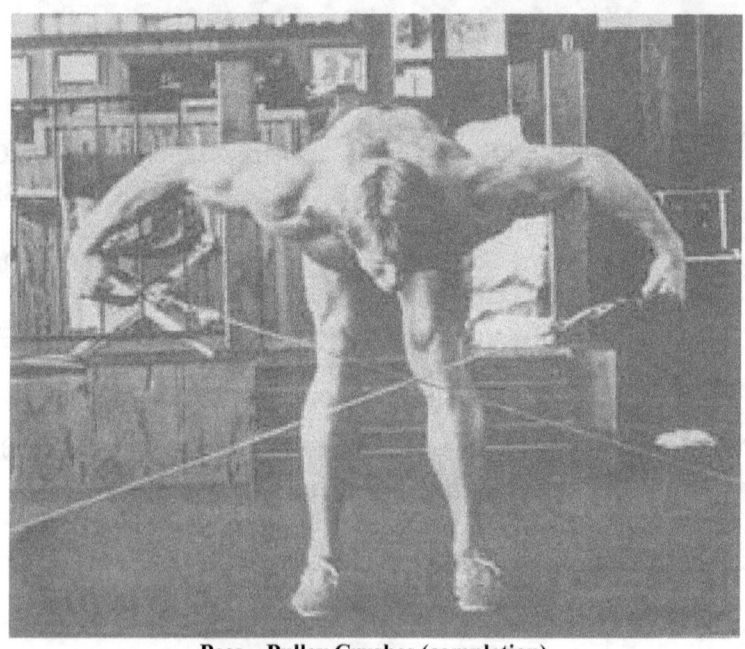

Pecs – Pulley Crushes (completion)

19

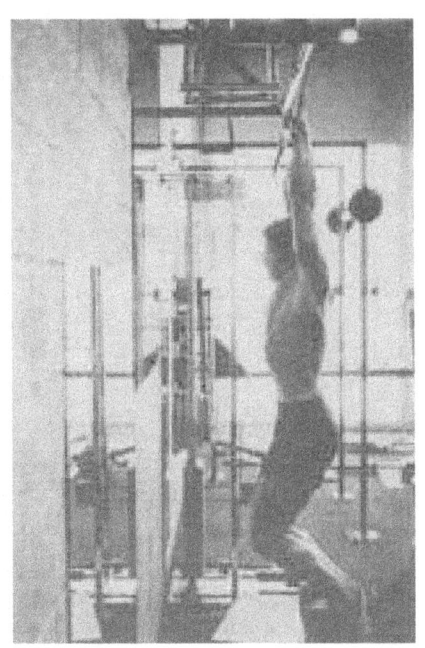

Abdominals – Hanging Knee Up (start)

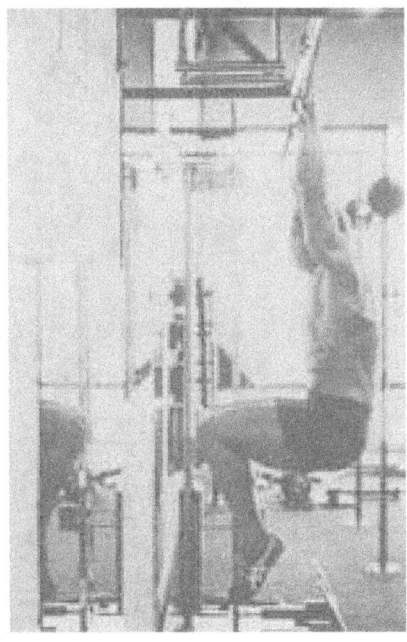

Abdominals – Hanging Knee Up (completion)

20

The Detailed Thigh

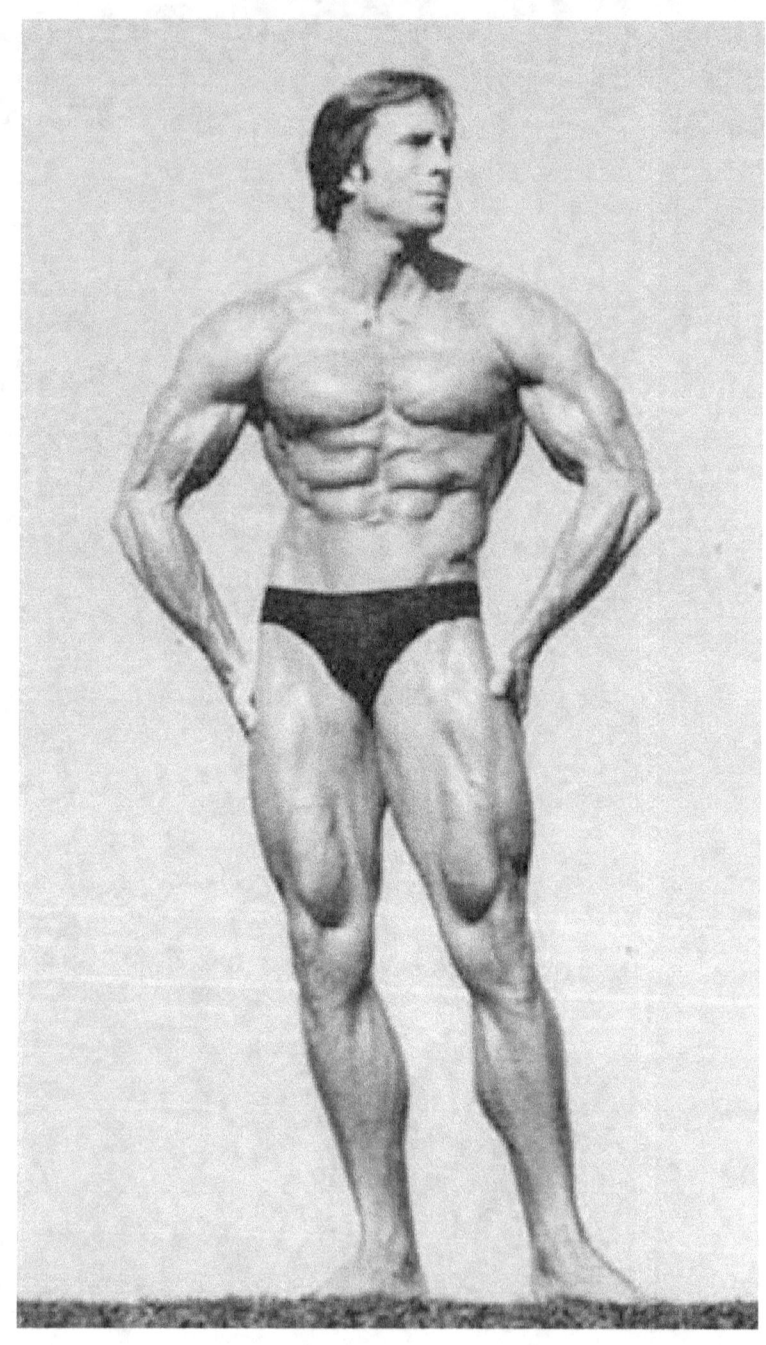

The Detailed Thigh

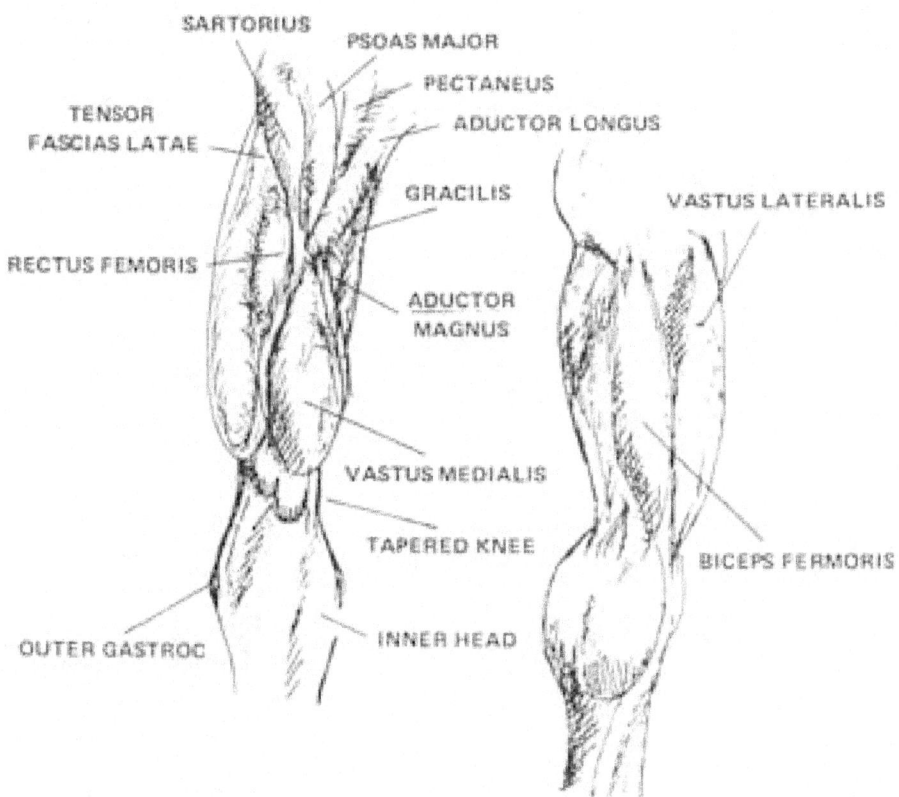

The key to impressive thigh development is the etching of each of the many small muscles of the frontal thigh. Then the trainee must balance the leg biceps with the frontal thigh.

SARTORIUS & PSOAS MAJOR – Hack Squat on toes with knees wide.

PECTANEUS, ADDUCTOR LONGUS-GRACILIS, ADDUCTOR MAGNUS – First half of parallel Hack Squat, Front Squat, Machine or Sissy Squat.

VASTUS LATERALIS & VASTUS MEDIALIS – Strive to achieve a balance between these two muscles, use parallel Hack Squat, Front Squat, and Leg Extensions.

LEG BICEPS – Balance and split the two heads with high repetition Leg Curls, Plié (wide, flat footed) Hack Squat. Separate the Vastas Lateralius from the leg biceps with a deep cut.

Train to develop each thigh muscle individually.

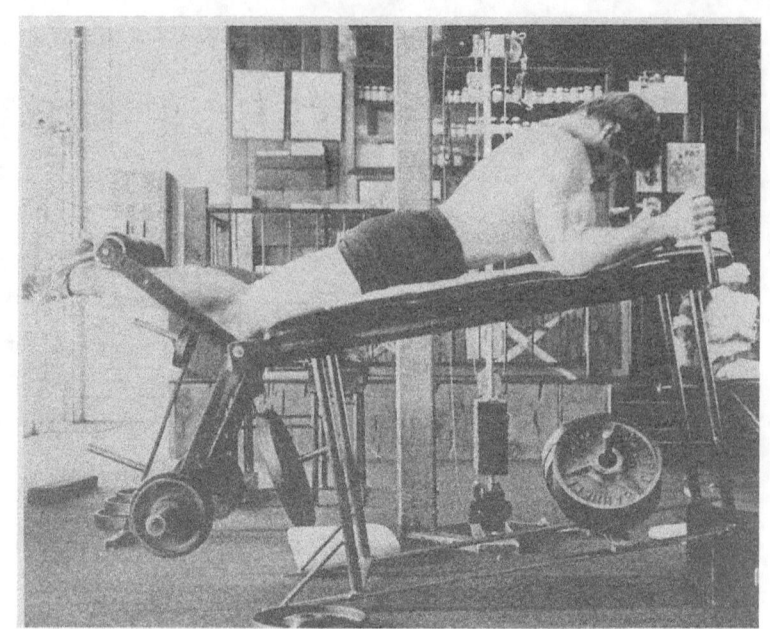

Thigh – Leg Curl (start) – note angle of table

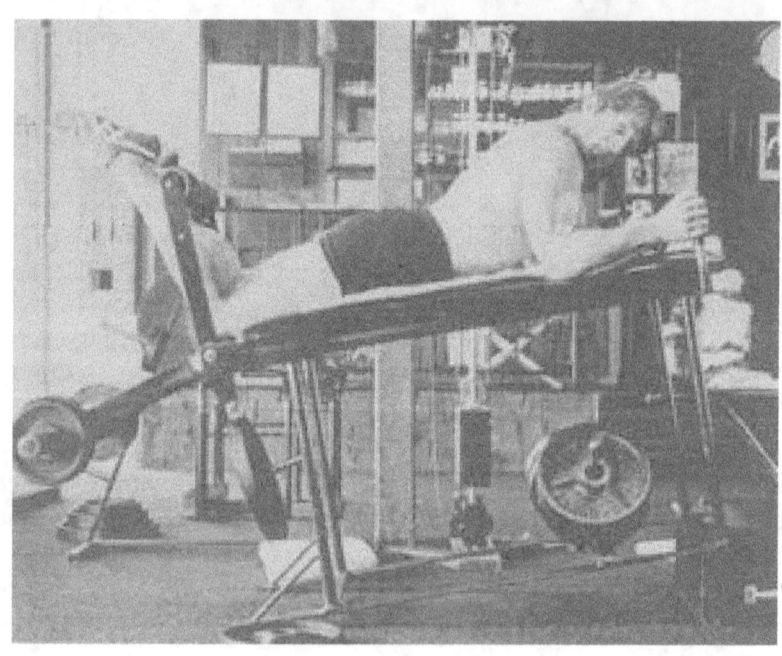

Thigh – Leg Curl (completion)

23

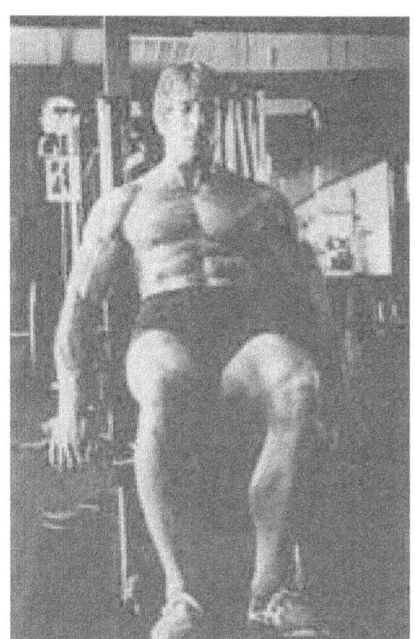

Thigh – Hack Machine Squat (start)

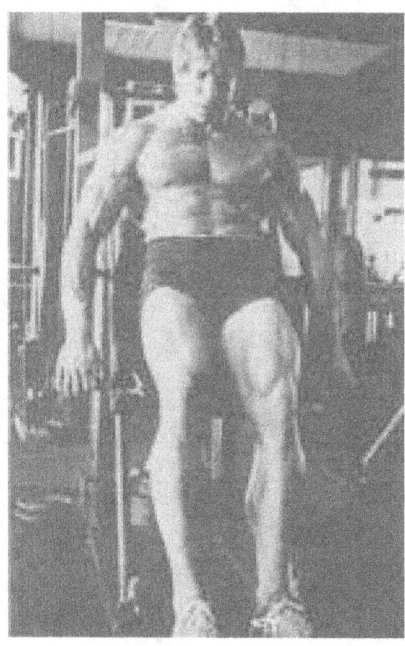

Thigh – Hack Machine Squat (completion) – note knees remain unlocked

The Symmetrical Arm

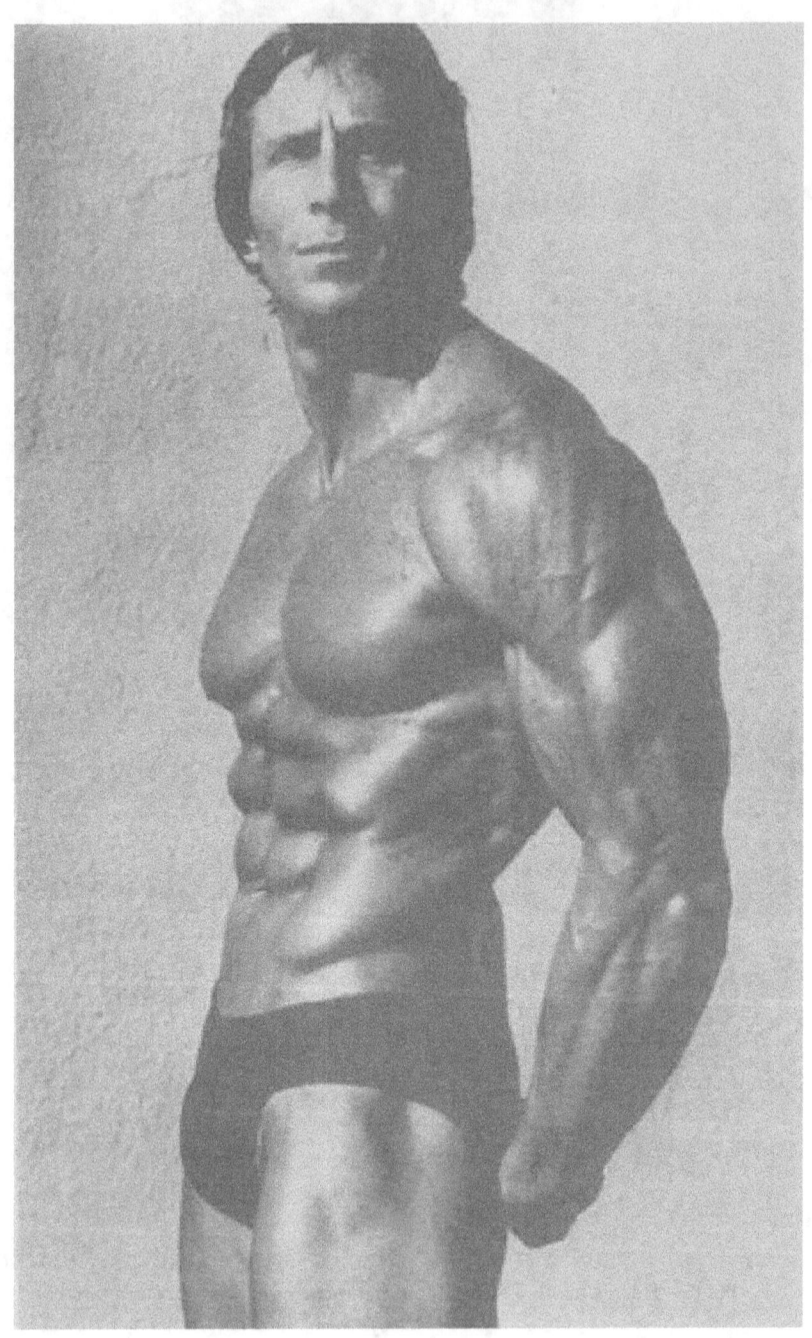

The Symmetrical Arm

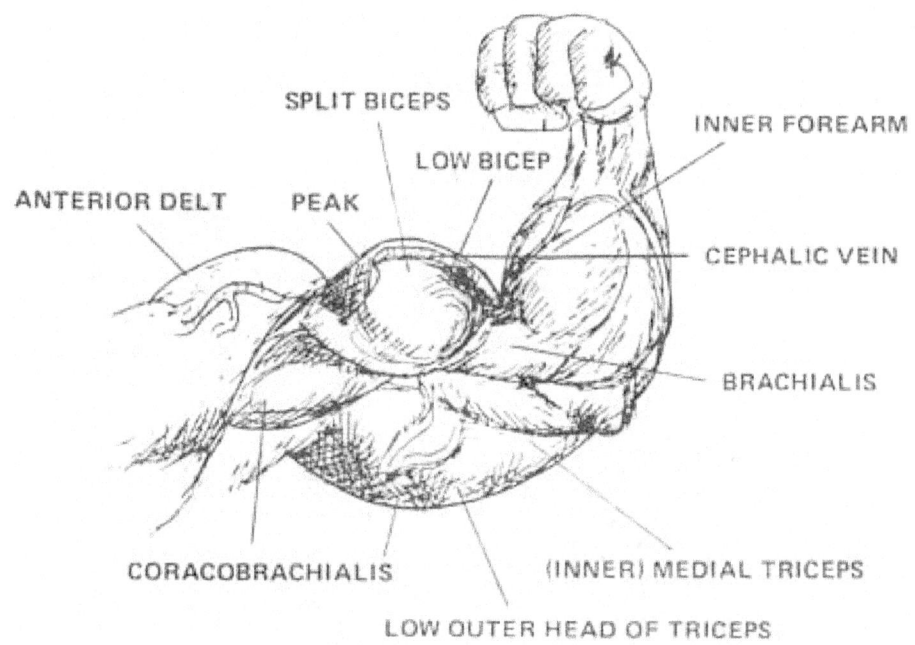

Remember, a proportionate arm means more than biceps & triceps. Seek equilibrium for all the upper arm muscles.

SPLIT BICEPS – (Biceps Brachii) Strict Curl, Incline Curl with continuous tension and peak contraction.

PEAK – Concentration Curls, Spider Curls, Cable Curls.

LOW BICEP – Preacher Curl, bottom half of all curling movements, D.B. Preacher Curl, Spider Curl.

LOW TRICEPS – Triceps pull on long pulley cable, full extension of triceps on all exercises, Pressdowns.

BRACHIALIS – Reverse Preacher Curl with Diametric Bar Reverse Curls.

CORACOBRACHIALIS – Bench Press, Close Grip Bench Press, Close Grip Press Behind Neck, Standing French Press.

CEPHALIC VEIN – Drag Curls, Crucifix Curls, Wide Grip Strict Curl, Close, Wide Preacher Curl.

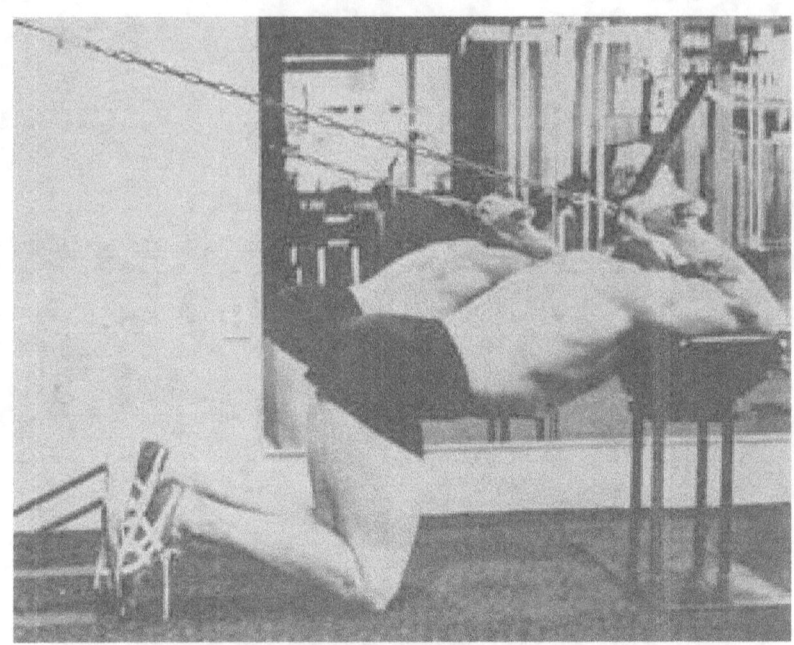

Triceps – Long Cable Pulley Extension (start)

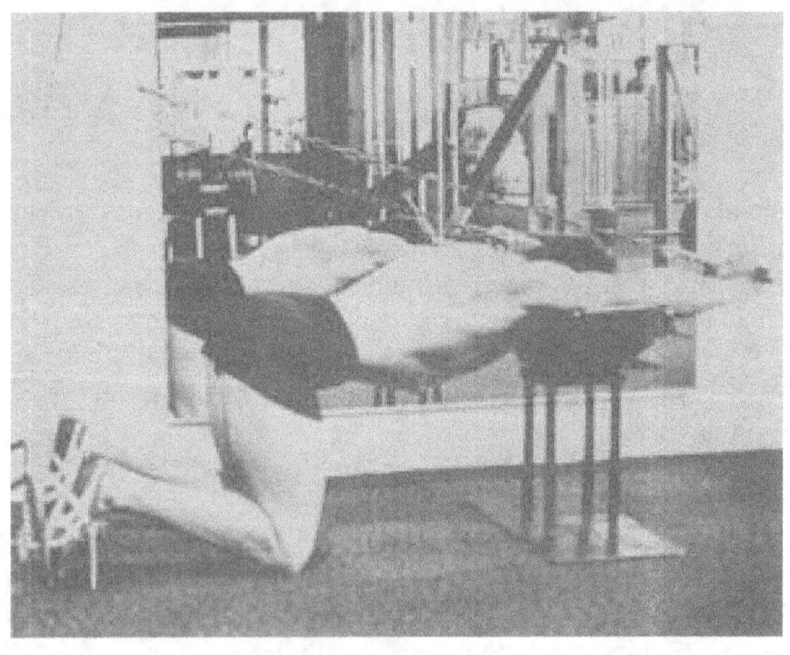

Triceps – Long Cable Pulley Extension (completion)

27

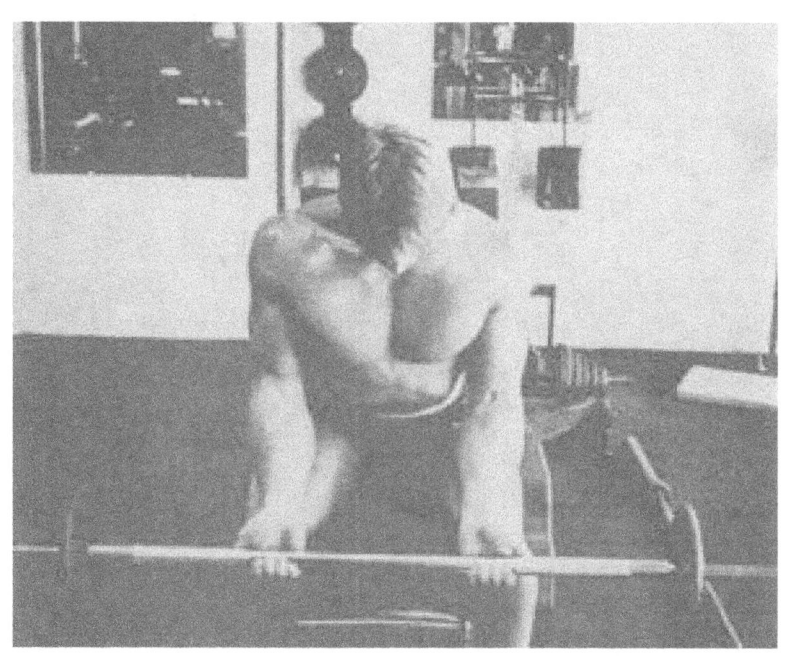

Forearms – Wrist Curl (start of movement)

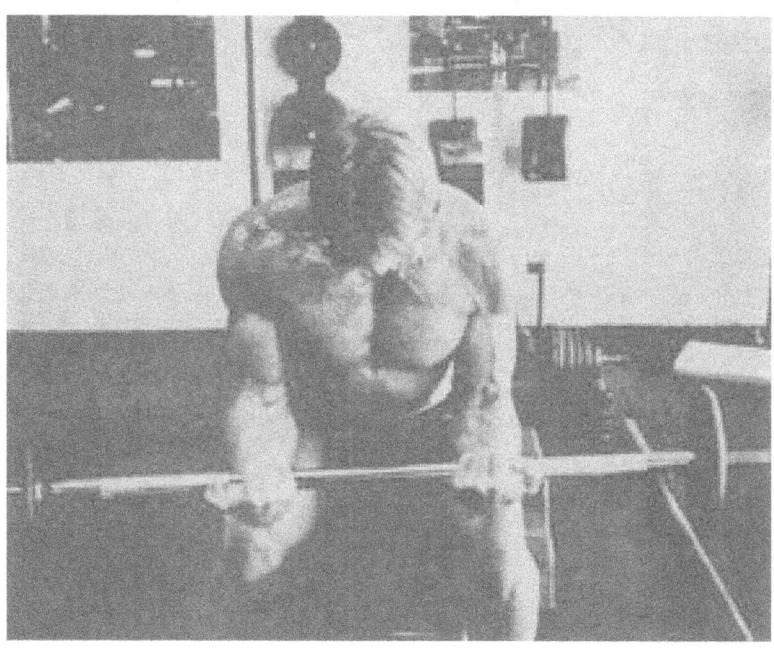

Forearms – Wrist Curl (completion of movement) – note false grip

28

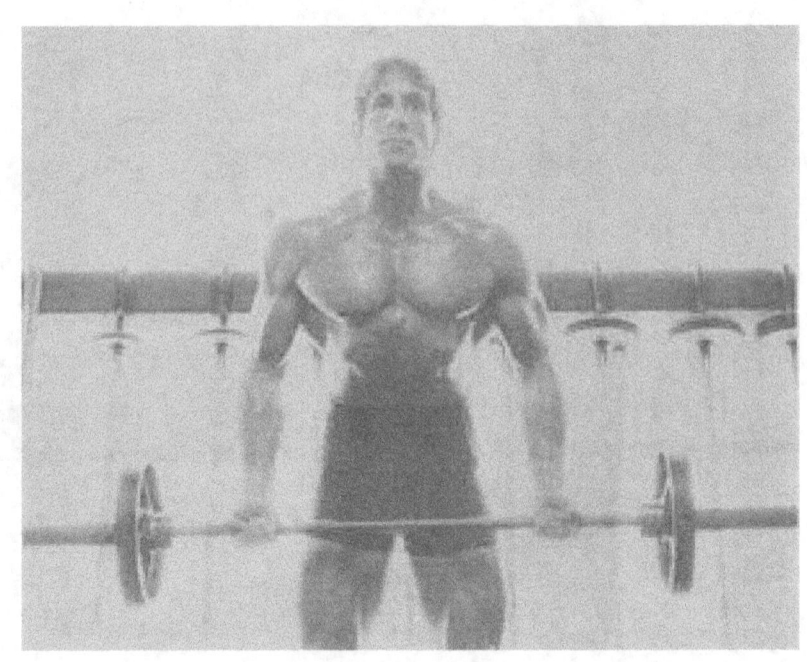

Biceps – Strict Curl (start of movement)

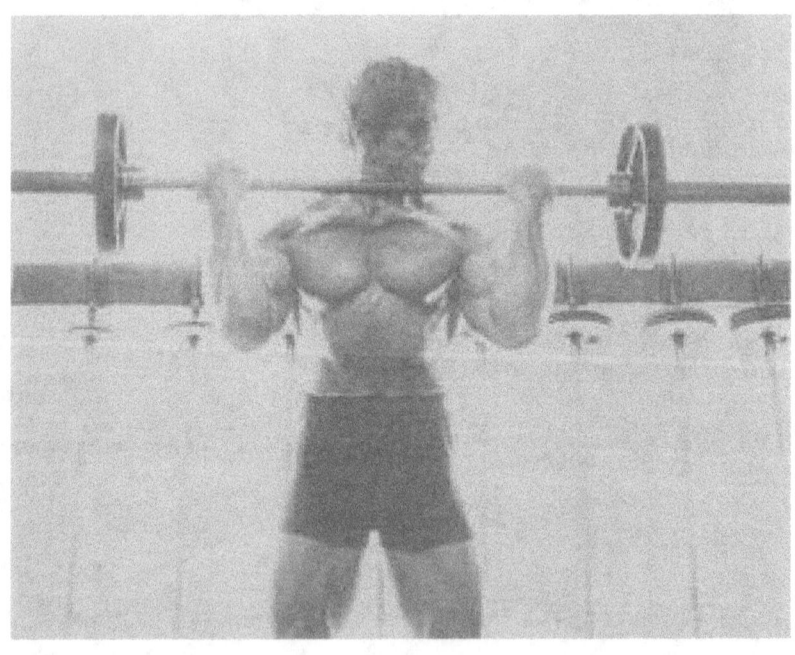

Biceps – Strict Curl (completion of movement)

The Total Deltoid

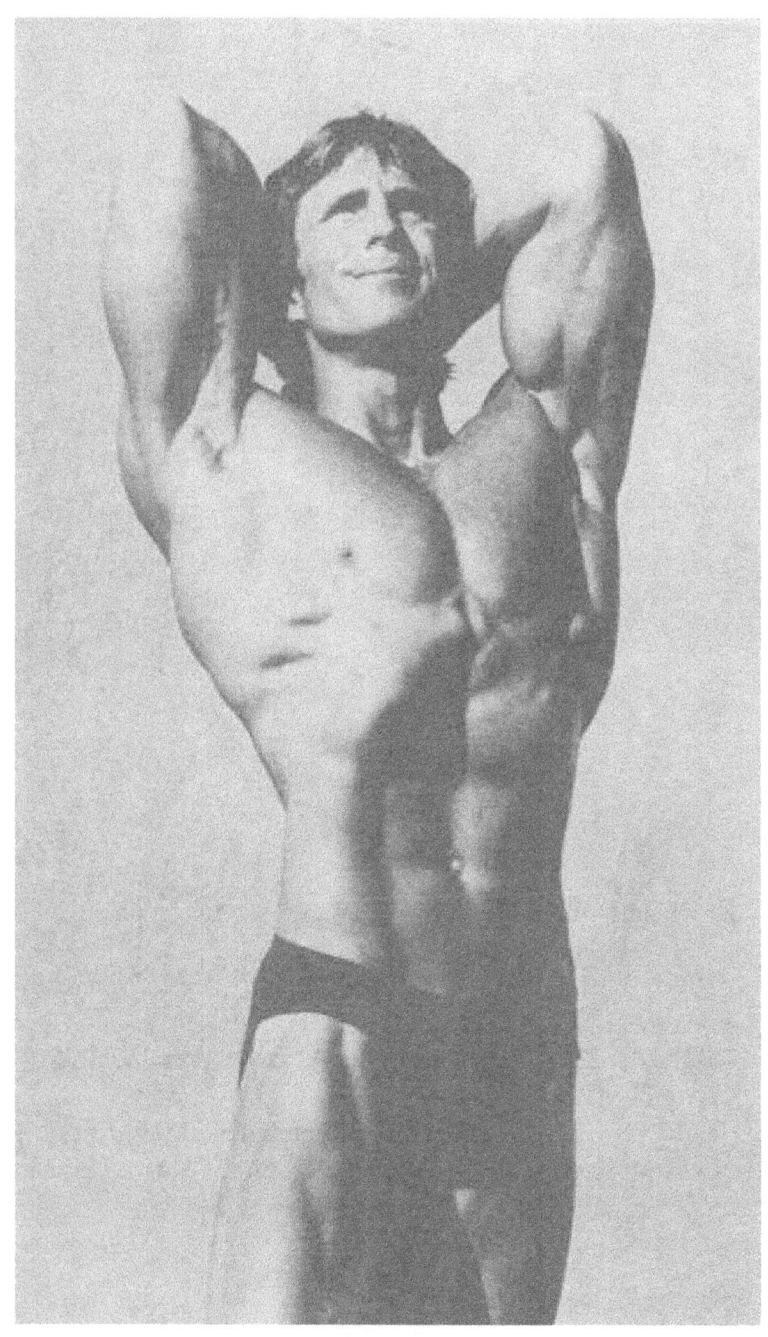

The Total Deltoid

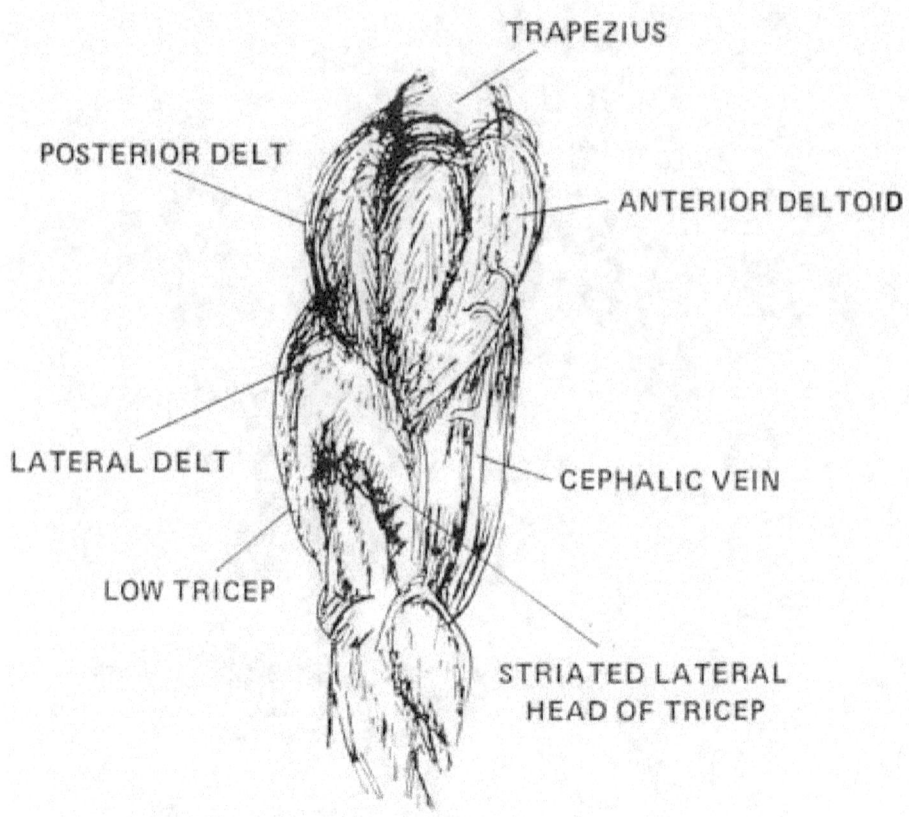

The three heads of the deltoid must be perfectly balanced with special stress on the lateral and posterior heads.

POSTERIOR DELTOID – Bent over laterals, bent over cable laterals, lying face down laterals on incline bench, press behind neck.

LATERAL DELTOID – Standing lateral raise, press behind neck, cable laterals, wide grip upright rows.

ANTERIOR DELTOID – Pressing movements, close grip upright rows, bench press on incline all forms of bench press. This is the easiest head to develop.

Train accordingly.

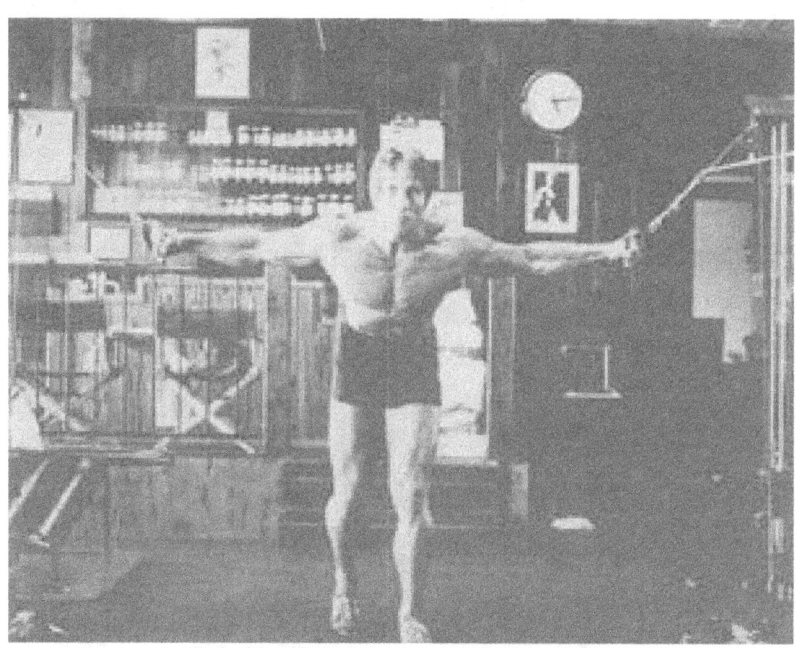

Deltoids – Bent-over Lateral Raise (start)

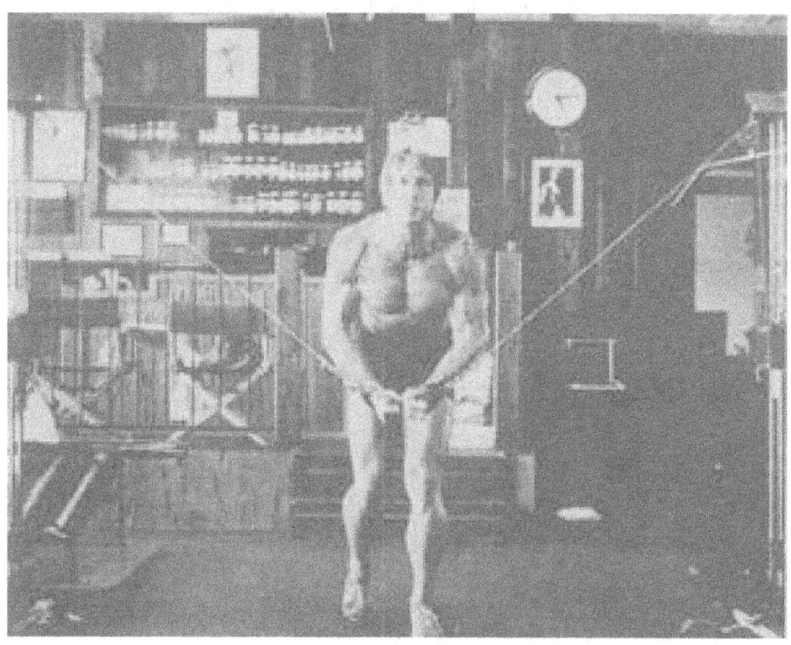

Deltoids – Bent-over Lateral Raise (completion)

32

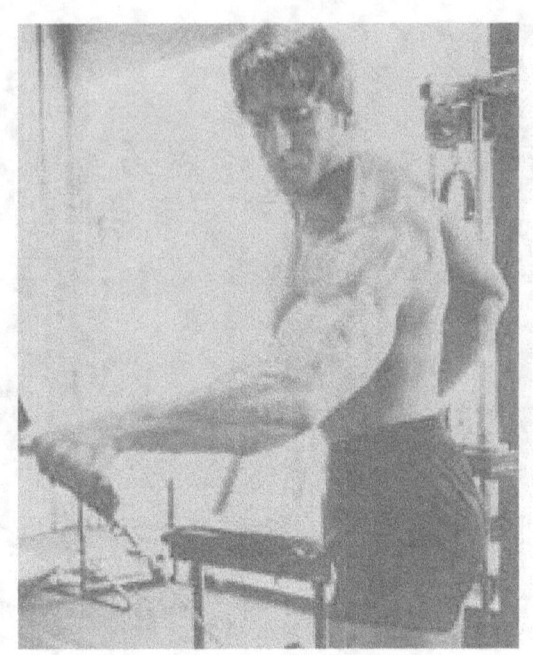

Deltoids – One Arm Cable Raise

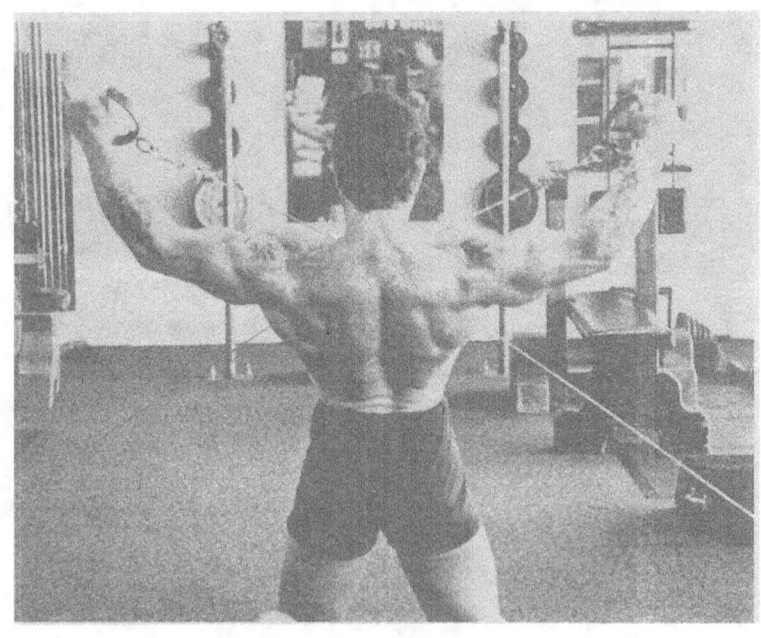

Deltoids – Two Arm Cable Raise

33

The Proportioned Calf

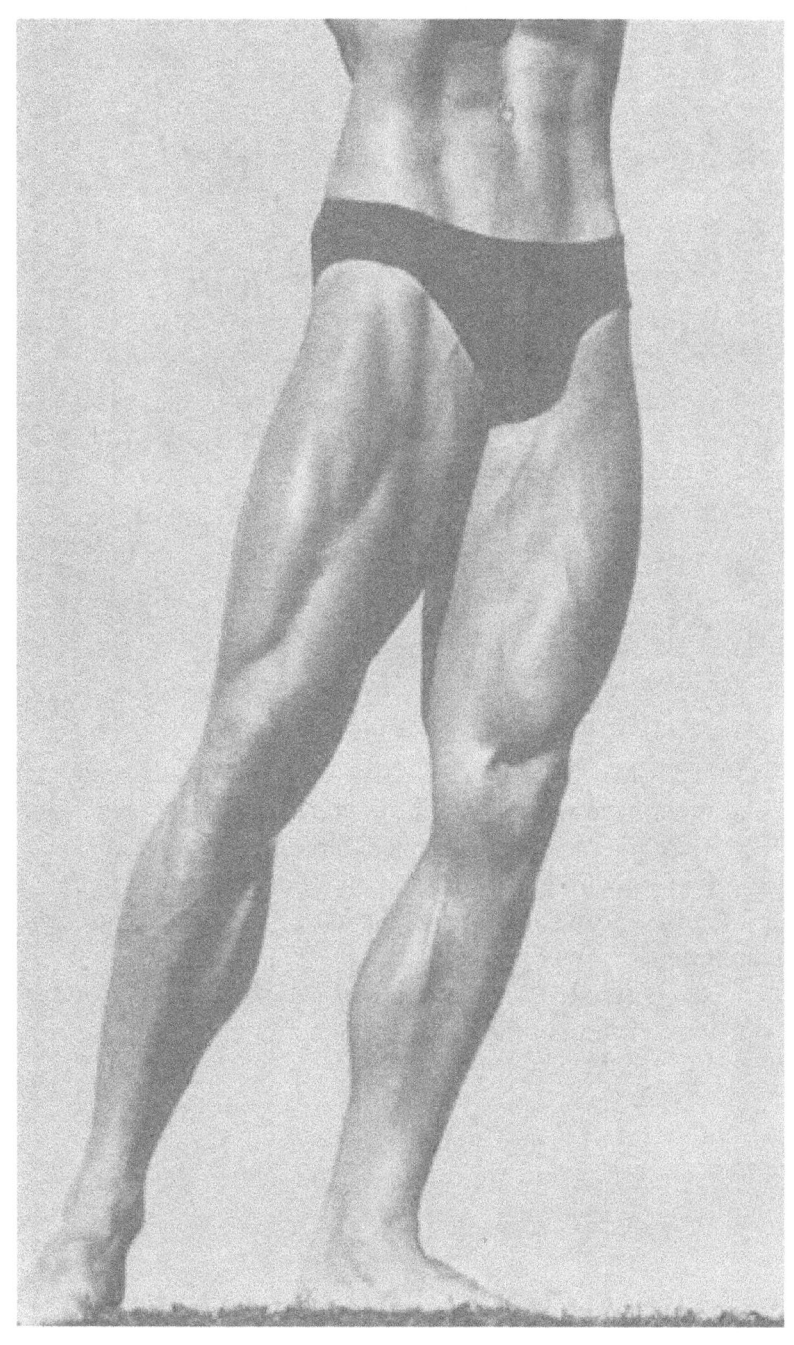

The Proportioned Calf

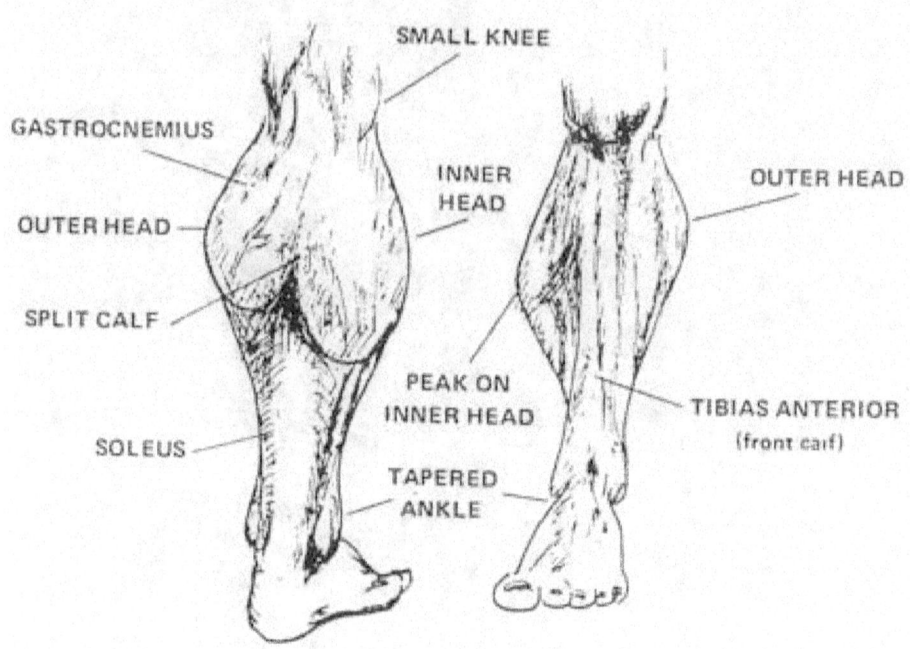

GASTROCNEMIUS PEAK – Press Machine Raise and Calf Raise working inner head with total contraction.

INNER HEAD – Toe Raise with heel close and toes wide.

SOLEUS – Seated raise, full stretch on all calf raises.

SPLIT CALF – Division of two heads of gastrocnemius achieved by peak contraction and continuous tension (via stretch).

TIBIAS ANTERIOR- (Frontal Calf) Raise of toes lying or sitting with feet off floor, curling of the toes to total contraction.

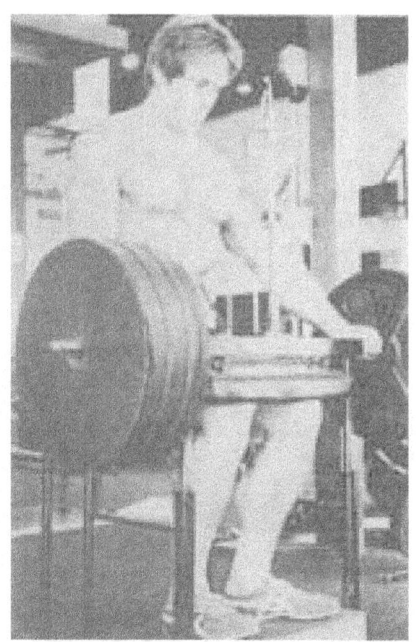

Calves – Seated Calf Raise (start)

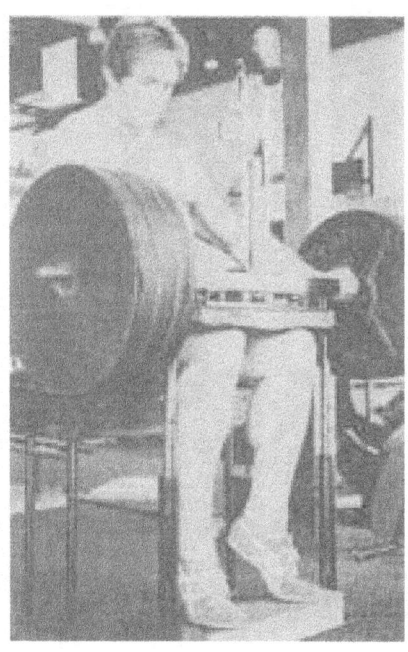

Calves – Seated Calf Raise (completion)

The Balanced Back

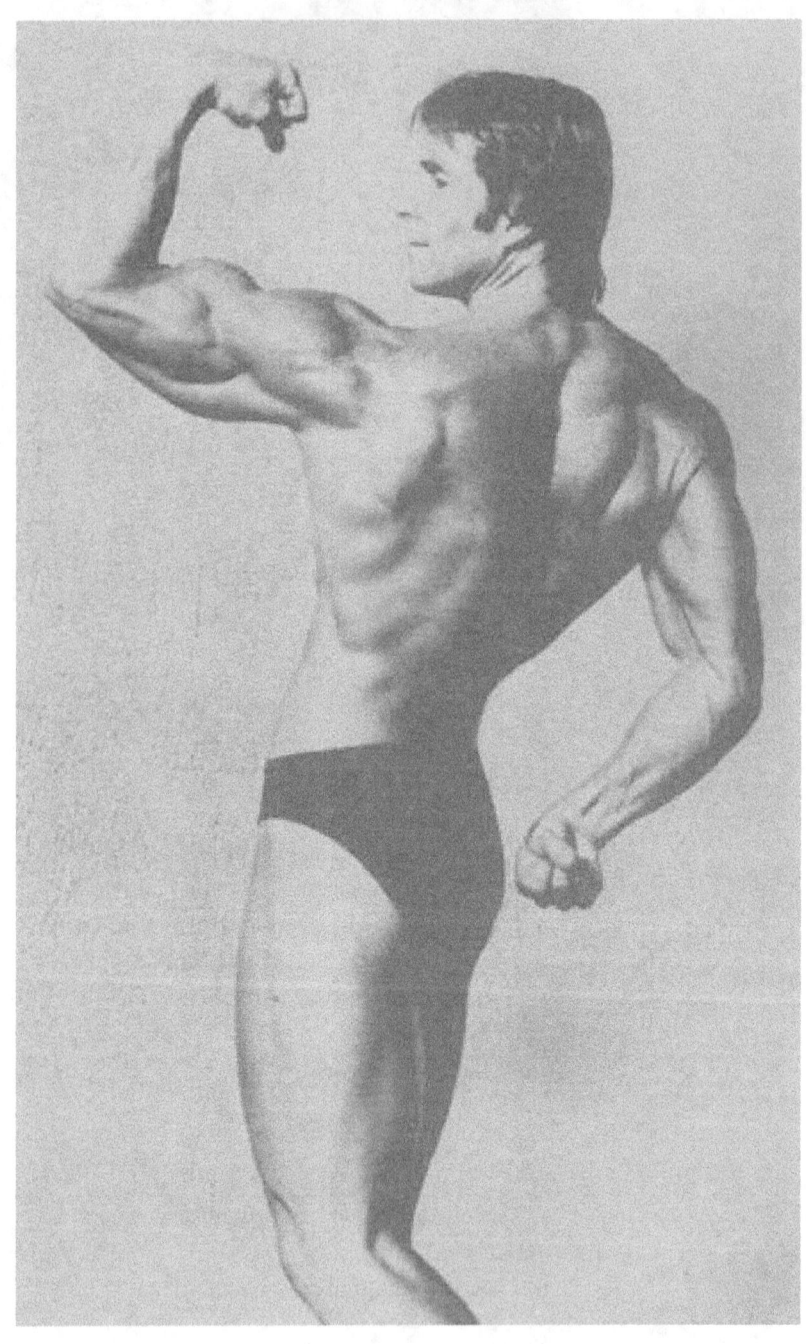

The Balanced Back

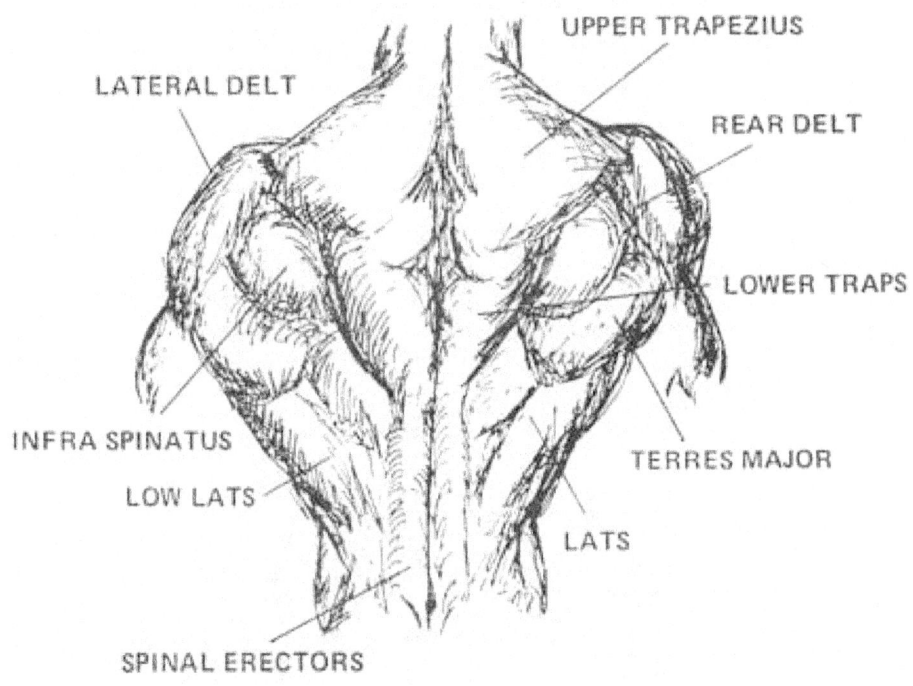

Although lumped together under the heading of lats, the back really consists of many muscles that must be carefully balanced.

TRAPEZIUS – Upright rowing, shrugs-be careful not to overdevelop.

REAR DELT – Bent over laterals, bent over cable laterals, rowing motions, press behind neck.

INFRA SPINATUS – Wide chins, long cable pulley rows, lat machine pull downs, barbell rowing.

TERRES MAJOR – UPPER LATISSIMUS – LOW LATISSIMUS – These three muscles tie in and can be worked similarly. Short cable pulley row, close grip bent over rows, one dumbbell rows.

SPINAL ERECTORS – Hyperextension, stiff legged dead lift, good mornings.

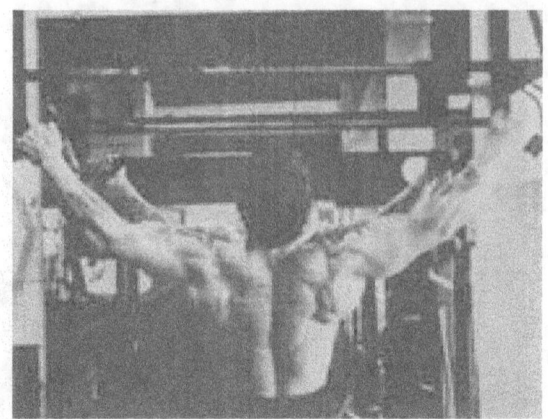
Back – Wide Grip Chins

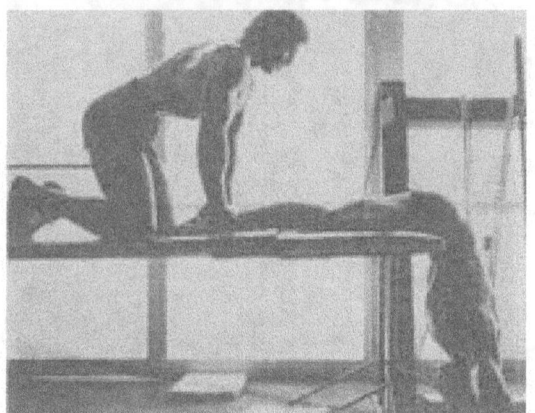
Lower Back – Hyperextension (start)

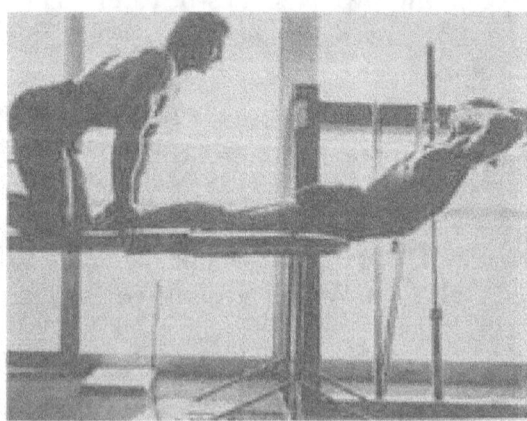
Lower Back – Hyperextension (completion)

Gaining Weight Proportionately

There is definitely a special method to adding muscle density. During this endeavor, the muscle (sarcoplast) and the muscle environment (sarcoplasm) ratio must be nearly equal. This means you must keep the ingestion of high quality, muscle building protein and complex carbohydrate at a higher than pre-contest level. Prior to a contest, when the diet is void of any significant carbohydrate level, the quantity of sarcoplasm is greatly diminished, which obviously causes the muscle girth to decrease proportionately. Unfortunately a high sarcoplasm content can cover up muscularity, so it is a necessary evil to reduce muscle size slightly, before a contest. But during a period of time when you are trying to gain size you must sacrifice some muscularity, but never to the point where your abdominals disappear. The off-season is a time for constructive training, not a time to get fat. Here is a diet I've used successfully to put on symmetrical muscle size and still maintain some muscularity and shape. Remember protein and more protein is the building block of human muscle.

Breakfast
3 Eggs-soft boiled
1 Orange or Apple
6 oz Cottage Cheese (raw)
4 oz Chicken or Fish
3 Lipo 1000 mg (Choline & Inositol)
10 Amino Acid Tablets
10 One Gram Liver Tabs
5 Energy Oils
1 Mega Multivitamin

Mid Morning
Protein Drink
3 heaping tablespoons Egg White Protein
2 Raw Eggs
8 oz Raw Certified Milk (non fat)
2 Enzymes Tablets
5 One Gram liver Tabs
5 Amino Acid Capsules
2 E (400 I.U.'s)

Lunch
8 oz Broiled Chicken or Fish
4 oz Cottage Cheese (raw)
10 One Gram Liver Tabs
10 Amino Acid Capsules
5 Energy Oils
2 B complex
2 E (400 I.U.'s)
2 C (500 mg's-Rose Hips)
3 Lipo 1000

One Hour Before Workout
Protein Drink same as Mid-Morning
2 Enzymes
5 Energy Oils
1 500 mg Niacin

Dinner
8 oz Broiled Chicken or Fish
Mixed Green Salad with Apple Cider Vinegar and Extra Virgin Olive
Oil dressing
5 One Gram Liver Tabs
5 Amino Acid Capsules

Application of Master Step Training

The intent of this book is to have you looking your symmetrical best the day of your most important contest, not one day, one week or one month later. For the best competitive success possible, plan one year ahead to be ready two weeks before your show. Things get frantic just prior to a show, so it is a big edge to have it all together just before. If you are too smooth and try to crash diet your way to muscularity, your cuts will not be deep and you will have to sacrifice too much size. Of course, each trainee responds quite differently in terms of metabolism, tolerance to a low-calorie diet and the ability to prepare for contest shape. With this in mind, let me give you a general outline for the entire contest year.

I. Master Step 12-9 Months Prior

A. Specialize on your most glaring weaknesses.
B. Go from 5-10 pounds (only!) over contest weight on the gain weight diet.
C. Train as heavy as possible with good strict form.
D. Use slightly lower repetition counts.

II. Master Step 8-4 Months Prior

A. Balance the work load to all body parts, but still keep a slight emphasis on your weaknesses.
B. Go to a moderate-low carbohydrate diet and bring your body weight back down gradually to within 5 pounds of contest shape. (Note: You should plan to enter the contest at least 5 pounds heavier than the previous year.)
C. Pick your training tempo up.
D. Use moderate weight and less rest between sets.

III. Master Step 3-2 Months Prior

A. Work every body part with near equal intensity.
B. Use the Master Pre-Contest diet detailed in "Total Muscularity": lower calories.
C. Train in a frenzy! Almost no rest between sets. Seek maximum burn and pump.
D. Start an aerobic program of thirty minutes 4-5 times per week. Use a treadmill or stationary bicycle for this purpose.

IV. Master Step Month Prior

A. Use this time to bring lagging body parts to contest shape so the entire body has balanced muscularity.
B. Stay on pre-contest diet.
C. Decide instinctively the quantity of reps you need to get muscular. For example, sometimes I use as many as 50 reps to cut my thighs up.
D. Don't do as much work as you have been doing up to this point, but train harder (more intensely).
E. Practice posing each day. Select 6-8 poses only, memorize them precisely and PRACTICE.

Balancing the Entire Physique

Now you have an outline for your quest for symmetry. You should have a clear picture of your physique and your goals. Remember, "natural" symmetry comes under the heading of special gifts. Yet, "knowledge is power." The ability to apply oneself 100% is also a special gift, but it is attainable by any who are willing to exercise the necessary discipline and make the appropriate sacrifices. This ability of total dedication belongs in some measure to the arts as well as sciences. It cannot, in the strict sense, be acquired by study alone.

You should use this book as a tool. I have attempted to anticipate your every need, and your every question in regard to that magical quality of physique I term symmetry. Sit down and blue print your training for the next year. Set realistic goals for yourself. Yet, keep this in mind, "A man's reach should exceed his grasp, or what's a heaven for?" Train Big!

Make a list of your strong points. Now, make a second list of your weaker body parts. Be objective! Don't spare yourself. You have been shown within these covers how to accentuate the lagging areas of your physique. No matter how slow your progress give this course a fair chance. Stress those slow to develop areas. Soon they will be up to par. True quality muscle always comes slowly. Train for quality and proportion. Welcome to the NEW BREED of bodybuilding.

Training for Detail

Finally, to acquire a totally symmetrical physique you must pay special attention to even the most minute details of each muscle group. Concentration is the key. Keep a mental picture of how you want each muscle to eventually look as you train it. Although the details I will discuss are not readily obvious in all cases, they can add greatly to the overall picture that the New Breed of bodybuilder strives to create.

One of the most eye-catching details that can enhance your entire physique is the thick cephalic vein that runs from the deltoid down through the middle of the two heads of the biceps and finally into the forearm. The more pronounced and outstanding you can make this vein, the more impressive your arm will look. Some trainees are blessed with an amazing amount of vascularity naturally. Others must train and diet to attain this important quality.

There are three movements that have proven especially effective in bringing out the cephalic vein. Crucifix curls are the first. You may do this movement seated or on an incline. Your palms must face outward (away from the body). Use a slightly less than locked (or "cocked") wrist. Wide grip barbell drag curls are also a fine delineator of the cephaelic. Use a thumbs under (false) grip and make sure to keep the bar in contact with your body throughout the movement. Dumbbell preacher curls with elbows held as close as possible are also effective in acquiring this important detail.

The forearms are often neglected totally. If they are trained at all they are worked by doing a few sets of wrist curls. This exercise works only the inner forearm. Very few bodybuilders are perceptive enough to seek equal development of the outer forearms. You can achieve this by adding reverse wrist curls, reverse preacher curls, reverse grip drag curls or plain standing reverse curls.

Similarly the outside of the calf is also left out of the average trainee's workouts. This area of the calf can look most impressive when viewed from the side. As mentioned before the seated raise affects this area directly. Other types of toe raises can be done in a pigeon-toed position to emphasize the outer calf. Also the addition of a few sets of donkey or other raises with the feet about 14"-16" inches apart and toes pointed in while keeping both knees touching will be effective. Try to get a full stretch even in this awkward position. It will help equalize the heads of the calf and spread the muscle wider.

Again, the erectors are a very important, oft-neglected area. Remember these twin muscles can be developed to the point of striated muscularity. Flex them forcibly at the completion of each hyperextension, dead lift, or good morning. The rear trapezius is another impressive detail when seen from the back. The bent over lateral raise is the finest movement for working this area. You may do this exercise seated with chest on knees, standing with the head supported or with cables, drawing the elbows back as far as possible when working the lats with pulldowns, or rowing motions.

The next detail of the physique that is most neglected is the inner thigh. There are a wide variety of exercises to bring out the many small muscles of the inner thigh. Squats or hack squats done with the feet spread wide at a 90° angle to the body are an effective way to hit this detail. Squeeze the thighs together against resistance as in the seated cable squeeze. This is perhaps the best movement to isolate this muscle group. Sit on a low bench with the soles of the feet together and the knees spread wide. Take a cable handle in each hand and brace the wrists against the outstretched knees with a false grip (thumbless) grip. Unlock the wrist to insure minimal usage of the arms. This is the key. Make sure to bring the unlocked wrists together without using the arm or pectorals. Concentrate on using the muscles of the inner thigh only. It is the small details of the physique that can make the difference between winning and losing. Train for detail and symmetry will surely follow.

The Famous Master Diets

The Master Diet: Level One

This is a diet designed for those of our students who have difficulty sticking to a low calorie diet. We prefer this type of food plan because intensive exercise such as we recommend increases the body's need for fuel. While in this diet you must restrict your carbohydrate intake to 40 grams (or preferably less) per day. This can easily be done by calculating the carbohydrate gram content in each food you eat. You will notice that some foods are high in carbohydrate and must be avoided. By using the attached list of carbohydrate values you can make sure you do not exceed the maximum limit of 40 grams per day. You may eat all the meat, pure fat (i.e. certified raw butter) and moderate amounts of most vegetables, certified raw cheese, and fertile eggs that you may wish. This means you can easily plan satisfying meals that will not leave you hungry. If you follow this diet exactly, you should lose 7-14 pounds per month. Remember restrict your carbohydrate intake to 40 grams, no more. The only way a person loses excess subcutaneous fat is through diet and exercise. Will power is the key. Stick to it! Check the maximum definition diet (for the final step) for your supplement list.

*Carbohydrate gram counters are available at most book stores and drug stores. Keep one of these small books with you until you memorize most of the food values.

Food	Serving Size	Carbohydrate Grams
Milk		
Whole Milk	8 oz.	11.8
Ice Cream	½ pint	14.8
Cheese		
Cheese	1 oz.	0.5
Cottage Cheese	1 rounded tbsp.	1.3

Food	Serving Size	Carbohydrate Grams
Fats		
Bacon	3 strips	0.0
Butter	1 tbsp.	0.0
French Dressing	1 tbsp.	1.9
Margarine	-----	0.0
Salad Oil	-----	0.0
Mayonnaise	1 tbsp.	0.2
Eggs		
1 egg	-----	0.73
Meat		
Bologna	2 slices	1.0
Frankfurter	1	1.9
Hash	1 serving	7.0
Chicken, Turkey, Ham, Veal, Beef, Lamb, Pork	1 serving	0.0
Nuts		
Mixed	10-15	3.0
Fish		
Oysters	4-6	1.2
Shrimp	5-6	0.5
Vegetables		
Asparagus	6 stalks	2.0
Beans, Green	½ cup	2.0
Beans, Lima	½ cup	23.5
Beet Greens	½ cup	5.6
Broccoli	½ cup	6.2
Brussels Sprouts	6	6.2
Cabbage	⅔ cup – cooked	5.3
Carrots	1 large	9.3
Cauliflower	4 oz.	3.4
Celery	2 stalks	1.9
Corn	1 ear	20.0
Cucumber	½	4.0
Eggplant	½ cup – cooked	5.6
Kale	½ cup – cooked	7.2
Lettuce	5 leaves	0.9
Lettuce	¼ head	1.8
Okra	6 pods	19.0
Onions	2-3 small	10.3
Green Peas	½ cup	17.7
Green Peppers	1	5.7
Potatoes	1 small	19.1
Spinach	½ - cooked	3.2

Food	Serving Size	Carbohydrate Grams
Squash	½ cup	7.1
Tomatoes	1 medium	0.4
Turnips	½ cup	7.1
Catsup	1 tbsp.	4.8
Tomato Juice	1 cup	4.3
Fruit		
Apples	1 large	22.4
Apricots	2-3	12.9
Avocado	½	5.1
Banana	1 small	23.0
Strawberries	10 large	8.1
Other Berries	⅔ cup	15.1
Cantaloupe	½ melon	6.9
Grapefruit	½ small	10.1
Grapes	22	16.7
Lemons	1 medium	8.7
Orange	1 small	11.2
Orange Juice	½ cup	12.9
Peach	1 medium	12.0
Pear	1 medium	15.8
Pineapple	½ cup	13.7
Plums	3 medium	12.9
Rhubarb	1 cup	3.8
Watermelon	1 wedge, about 10 oz.	22.0
Canned Fruit		
Cherries	½ cup	20.0
Cranberry Sauce	1 tbsp.	10.2
Pineapple in syrup	1 slice	21.1
Dried Fruit		
Apricots	4-6	20.0
Prunes	2-3	21.3
Cereals		
Cornflakes	1 cup	18.0
Oatmeal	½ cup – cooked	13.0
Puffed Rice	¾ cup	8.6
Shredded Wheat	1 biscuit	24.0
Spaghetti, Macaroni	½	14.8
Noodles	½ cup	14.8
White Rice	½ cup – cooked	15.8
Tapioca	1 tbsp.	12.9
Flour Meal		
Corn Meal	½ cup	15.7
Cornstarch	1 tbsp.	10.0

Food	Serving Size	Carbohydrate Grams
Bread		
White	1 slice	13.0
Rolls	1 parker house	16.0
Crackers	1 – 2"x3"	7.0
Graham Crackers	1	7.0
Sugars		
Honey	1 tbsp.	15.0
Jam	1 level tbsp.	14.2
Jellies	1 level tbsp.	13.0
Brown Sugar	1 tbsp.	10.5
Granulated Sugar	1 tbsp.	5.0
Syrup – table blends	1 tbsp.	14.8
Miscellaneous		
Bouillon Cubes	2	4.7
Coca	2 tbsp.	3.0
Gelatin Dessert powder	1 tbsp.	5.3
Beverages		
Beer	12 oz. bottle	12.0
Sodas – various	8 oz. bottle	21.6
Gin and Rum	1 jigger	0.0
Crème de menthe	1 cordial glass	6.0
Whiskey	-----	0.0
Wine, Red	1 wine glass	0.5
Wine, Port	1 wine glass	4.0
Sherry	1 wine glass	2.4

The Master Definition Diet: Level Two

This diet is specially designed and not meant to be used for extended periods of time. To begin with, all carbohydrates must be removed from a maximum definition diet. This means all fruit, all vegetables, all salad greens and all milk products (cheeses, yogurt, ice cream milk and buttermilk). The only milk products that can be used are butter and cream. Any kind of meat, fish or fowl and eggs are the only foods permissible. You must, however, eat some carbohydrate every seven days because you will find that you will smooth out and veins and cuts will disappear. You will find also that you are not getting the pump you should and your strength will decrease. This is because a zero carbohydrate diet drains all the stored glycogen from the liver, and only carbohydrate will replenish it. But don't try to eat a small amount of carbohydrate each day. You will only find you are smoothing out. Do not use salt, it retains water. Other spices like pepper, garlic, and oregano are good because they stimulate enzyme production.

Breakfast:
    Eggs, No Limit
        Scrambled in butter
        Poached
        Boiled, Soft or Hard Sunnyside up-in butter
    Meat (no limit)
        Hamburger Patty
        Steak
        Chops, Lamb
        Liver
        Chicken Livers
        Kidney
        Brains

Lunch:
    Eggs (Cooked any way)
    Meat (Same as breakfast)
        Turkey
        Chicken
        Fish (fresh)
        Canned Tuna (6 oz. in water)
        Hamburger patty

Dinner:
        Same as breakfast and lunch
        Roasts (all kinds)
        *Tossed Green Salad if necessary to provide roughage consisting of ¼ head of lettuce, ¼ cucumber, 1 slice tomato, apple cider vinegar, safflower oil and spices.

✓ Never use salt! It only serves to retain water, and since the human body is 70% liquid, weight loss is slowed down to a standstill.

✓ Use garlic, pepper, mustard seed and oregano instead of salt. These spices actually increase enzyme production.

✓ Do not use ketchup or commercial meat sauces as they contain white sugar (sucrose) which translates to fat. Try Grey Poupon Dijon Mustard.

✓ Recommended Beverages: Rose Hips Tea as a natural diuretic, low sodium content diet drinks and purified water.

✓ Use certified raw butter whenever possible.

Pre-Contest Diet: Level Three

Muscularizing your physique must be a gradual process, taking anywhere from four to six months to accomplish. Those bodybuilders who bulk up 20-30 pounds and then starve to get definition the last six weeks before a show are the same people who complain about not having the necessary combination of size and muscularity the night of the contest. I maintain that the only way to achieve both size and muscularity, is to muscularize gradually; to use the levels approach in carbohydrate decrease.

I have broken the Master Diet down into three levels: For the first two months use a Low Carbohydrate diet, the third and fourth months, The Master Definition Diet and the last eight weeks before the contest, The Pre-Contest Diet. Simply stated, this plan is a gradual decrease in consumed carbohydrates: 40 grams at level one, 10-15 grams at level two and 0-5 at the pre-contest level.

In 1975, I was extremely muscular for the Mr. California contest in April. I started decreasing my carbohydrate consumption in January. After this contest, I continued decreasing my carbohydrate intake, but by the middle of May, I began gaining size on a nearly zero carbohydrate diet, so that by July at the American Bodybuilding Championships, I was bigger and more muscular than in April. Point: to increase muscularity and muscle size, plan your diet six months before the contest you are planning to win. Besides attaining the combination of size and muscularity, this diet will allow you ample time for physique preparation. You should be ready 30 days before the contest. In this way, you can devote your time during those last days preparing to give the best exhibition of your life, rather than worrying about losing one half inch on your arm or whether your abdominals will be cut up enough. I win physique contests because I plan ahead, I retain size with muscularity and I'm in top shape a day early. Now, doesn't this approach seem more effective?

Diet

Breakfast:	Lunch:	Dinner:
3 soft boiled eggs	1 can tuna packed in water	6 - 8 oz. fish
½ grapefruit		Supplements
supplements	supplements	

New Breed Supplements for Growth and Muscularity

To achieve increased muscle size and muscularity, it is important to increase your ingestion of food supplements as these supplements contain concentrated amounts of vital tissue building and muscularity producing nutritional elements, without necessitating the consumption of vast quantities of food which will ruin your hopes of attaining a small, wasp waist at the same time.

The key to determining the quality of the supplements you use is the source from which they are made. In all cases, the supplements you use must be derived from natural sources. Synthetic vitamins are never used by those people who have even the slightest understanding of nutrition. Take it from me, there is a vast difference between Ascorbic acid and Rose Hip not only in its source, but also in its effect on your plans to develop a championship phyique.

The New Breed of bodybuilder is dedicated to a scientific and intelligent physical pursuit, and as natural supplements represent the combination of the highest quality products, that is what you should strive to use.

This list of supplements is to be consumed with each meal with the exception that vitamin E will be substituted for iron at dinner, since these supplements cancel each other out when taken together. You must consume your supplements with each meal in order to increase your body's ability to withdraw nutrients from supplements. As it is, the body's efficiency of extracting nutrients as they pass through the digestive tract is anywhere from 30-50% effective. This is one reason for larger quantities of supplements taken throughout the day. Try to get your supplements in capsule form, as this may promote better assimilation by the body.

Total Supplementation Guide

Supplements per meal on levels I, II and III of the Master Diet.

3 Amino Acid Capsules-predigested protein for tissue growth
10 One gram Liver extract tablets-to increase muscular strength and endur-ance
10 Kelp-the natural way to increase your metabolism
3 Lipo capsules-contains choline and inositol to burn off subcutaneous fat and increase muscularity
2 HCL (hydrochloric acid) tablets-to improve protein digestion and utilization
3 Lecithin capsules-to burn the body's fat pockets and increase your skin tone
2 Calcium (4 calcium at bedtime)-to maintain calcium phosphorus bal-ance and tranquilize the nerves
1 500 mg. C-a natural diuretic
2* 400 I.U. E-increased endurance and muscle tone
1 100 mg. niacin-to improve vascularity
2 B complex capsules-provides necessary enzymes for carbohydrate combustion to create an energetic feeling when you hit the gym.
5 Germ Oil Capsules – male hormone precursor that facilitates tissue growth
*Substitute 3 iron tablets at dinner only.